LYSERGIC ACID DIETHYLAMIDE (LSD)
IN THE TREATMENT OF ALCOHOLISM

BROOKSIDE MONOGRAPHS

Publications of the Addiction Research Foundation
344 Bloor Street, West, Toronto 4, Canada

Under the general editorship of
P. J. GIFFEN, Department of Sociology, University of Toronto
R. E. POPHAM, Addiction Research Foundation

LYSERGIC ACID DIETHYLAMIDE (LSD) IN THE TREATMENT OF ALCOHOLISM

An Investigation of its Effects on
Drinking Behavior, Personality Structure,
and Social Functioning

REGINALD G. SMART, PH.D.

THOMAS STORM, PH.D.

EARLE F. W. BAKER, M.D., F.R.C.P.(C)

LIONEL SOLURSH, M.D., F.R.C.P.(C)

Brookside Monograph of the Addiction Research Foundation No. 6

PUBLISHED FOR THE ADDICTION RESEARCH FOUNDATION

BY UNIVERSITY OF TORONTO PRESS

Foreword

THE DISTINGUISHED PHYSIOLOGIST, A. J. Carlson, was noted for one question which he invariably addressed, in Swedish accents, to a young investigator who claimed to have made a discovery: "What is the evidence?" And, when presiding at a scientific meeting, his admonition to a garrulous reporter, "We are interested in your facts, Doctor, not your hypotheses," cleared the room of a volume of words and pointed out to the young scientist his first responsibility.

For the many types of alcoholism there are many treatments. The proponents of each claim it to be effective. A therapist, unconscious of the primary contribution of his personality, may believe that the success which follows his regimen is due to the formula. Unaware that the most important ingredient of his method, himself, cannot be prescribed by another, he advertises its virtues and cannot accept reports of its failure in other hands. He may lose his objectivity because his patients praise him and because of their tendency to tell him what pleases him. His published reports may be based on impressions and hypotheses rather than on substantial, controlled evidence.

When early experiments with a new drug reveal startling effects upon a particular illness, it is hailed as the answer to wide therapeutic needs. This was the experience with cortisone, twenty years ago. A small dose produced euphoria and freedom of movement in a patient who had been bedridden with rheumatoid arthritis. Immediately, it was hailed as the miracle drug and tested in a variety of clinical conditions for which no remedy had been found. Extravagant claims of success followed until the narrow limits of its usefulness were revealed by careful investigation.

It is also twenty years since it was discovered that lysergic acid diethylamide can produce emotional and behavioral changes in the mentally ill; and it was a natural consequence to administer it to patients whose problems in living led them to seek refuge in alcohol. Conclusions of success based upon uncontrolled experiments followed.

An objective study, by those who will coldly ask for facts, not only in relation to experiments carried out in their own institutions but also in reports published in scientific journals, should provide reliable evaluation of a form of treatment. The basic requirement is that results should be measured in a controlled environment, by clinicians trained in scientific research, or guided by those who have such experience. The authors of this Monograph enjoy that reputation. They have conducted a study, and analyzed its results. They have had conversations with others who have professed success in their particular therapy. They have carefully surveyed the literature and examined claims dispassionately. Their conclusions have been based on the question "What is the evidence?" These conclusions will not be invariably accepted, because a "fact" is an expression of judgment and not all evidence is free from personal opinion.

The reader is assured, however, that this careful appraisal of contemporary knowledge of the usefulness of lysergic acid diethylamide in the treatment of alcoholism has been prepared with the expressed purpose "not to argue that it has no effect, but solely to show that the Scottish verdict 'not proven' is the only one justified by the evidence."

G. H. ETTINGER, M.D.

Chairman,
Professional Advisory Board,
Addiction Research Foundation

Preface

IN 1962 AS A RESULT OF A GROWING NUMBER of clinical reports that LSD was of definite value in the treatment of the alcoholic, Dr. E. F. W. Baker approached the Addiction Research Foundation (A.R.F.) to see whether a study of the usefulness of LSD in the treatment of alcoholics could be made. After considerable discussion with Dr. J. D. Armstrong, formerly of the Clinical Division of the A.R.F., a plan was developed for the study, using volunteers from the Foundation's clinical services. A research grant was made to Dr. Baker, and the Research Division of the Foundation provided scientific advice about the design, the follow-up criteria, and the scheduling of patients. The staff of the Research Division, through Dr. Smart, were responsible for the pre- and post-treatment assessments, the conduct of follow-ups, and the analysis and reporting of the data. Dr. Storm helped with the planning of the study and with the data analyses and final report. Drs. Baker and Solursh administered the LSD, made the pre- and post-drug psychiatric assessments, and collaborated on the final report.

The present monograph, in addition to reporting the results of what is one of the first controlled trials of LSD as an adjunct to the treatment of alcoholism, is believed to be a departure from most previous studies in that an attempt is made to evaluate the utility of LSD and because primary interest is focused on its use with alcoholics. The literature relevant to the use of LSD in alcoholism treatment is brought together in order to evaluate the conclusions with scientific standards in mind. Several appraisals of LSD have been published: Unger, for example, reviewed the psychological effects of the drug up to 1962, Hoffer the psychological and therapeutic effects up to 1964, and Cohen the dangers of LSD as known in 1960. Such reviewers appear to accept the utility of LSD and therefore have been more concerned with the strategy of discovery than with the strategy of proof and none of them was especially concerned with alcoholism, although it would appear that the only current therapeutic indication for LSD is in the treatment of alcoholics.

In carrying out the LSD study and in preparing this report, the writers trespassed unconscionably on the time and patience of many tolerant people. Dr. J. D. Armstrong, then Medical Director, A.R.F., and Dr. G. Fraser, then Administrator of the A.R.F. Hospital are chief among them. They facilitated many of the inconvenient arrangements necessary to involve alcoholic patients in the study and provided advice and support at many junctures. Miss Gardner of the Toronto Western Hospital nursing service was responsible for nursing the patients after their LSD experience, and Miss Helen Lazarski of the A.R.F. nursing staff helped with many of the problems raised by the participation of Foundation patients. Mr. Richard Bennett and Mrs. Marnie Marley conducted the follow-up interviews which were time-consuming and frustratingly difficult to arrange. The authors are also indebted to the therapists and administrators of the A.R.F. clinical facilities who generously tolerated the disruptions in their work necessary to permit a properly controlled evaluation.

Special thanks should also go to Mr. Erich Polacsek of the A.R.F. Drug Archives for continually searching the LSD literature and for keeping us abreast of all current research on hallucinogens.

The editors of the Brookside Monograph series, Professor P. J. Giffen, and Mr. R. E. Popham, provided encouragement in the early stages of writing and critical appraisal in the later stages.

Dr. R. J. Gibbins, Dr. H. Kalant, and Dr. W. Schmidt of the A.R.F. Research Division read the manuscript and offered many helpful criticisms and suggestions. Dr. Kalant also generously made his considerable experience with the technical problems of drug evaluation research available to the investigators during the planning stages.

Miss Beryl Brown showed unusual forbearance in typing and retyping the several drafts of the report.

Parts of the material in Chapter 3 were reported in a paper by Smart and Storm in the Quarterly Journal of Studies on Alcohol, Vol. 25, pp. 333–38, 1964. Some of the material in Chapters 4 and 5 was reported in a paper by Smart, Storm, Baker, and Solursh in the Quarterly Journal of Studies on Alcohol, Vol. 27, pp. 469–82, 1966. These chapters have been extensively revised and enlarged for this monograph, but the earlier material is reproduced by permission of the Journal of Studies on Alcohol, Inc., New Brunswick, New Jersey.

R.G.S.
T.S.
E.F.W.B.
L.S.

Contents

LYSERGIC ACID DIETHYLAMIDE (LSD)
IN THE TREATMENT OF ALCOHOLISM

1. Discovery and Early Use of LSD

INTRODUCTION

THERAPEUTIC USE OF LSD represents one of the few radical developments in the treatment of alcoholism. Since the introduction of antabuse therapy by Jacobsen in 1951 and tranquilizers in 1954 the number of new therapies for alcoholism has been very small. This is not to say that new therapies are not needed. Improvement rates under all existing therapies are still only about 40 per cent (Bacon, 1963.) At first glance LSD seems to offer every advantage expected of a new therapy. It is inexpensive and easy to administer, and it is reported to be effective after only one administration. Early reports of its use with alcoholics have claimed improvement rates up to 94 per cent—based on reduced drinking and improved social stability. This percentage exceeds those for almost all known therapies for alcoholics and hence LSD therapy demands close attention and careful scrutiny. To date, we do not feel that the use of LSD has been given the analysis it deserves. For example, there appear to be no reviews of its use in therapy which are at once comprehensive and critical and a number of its adherents have an uncritical approach to its use. Its utility in the treatment of alcoholism has not been completely analyzed and interpreted, although it seems that this utility is taken for granted in some clinics.

One purpose of this monograph is to compile and synthesize existing knowledge about the effects of LSD on personality, social, and psychiatric variables and to examine the empirical warrant for its use in treating mental disorders. Special attention will be paid to an examination of its effectiveness in treating alcoholics. A second purpose is to report the results of a large-scale investigation of the effects of a single dose of LSD on drinking, social, and personality variables in alcoholics. To date, this is the first such

3

investigation employing control groups, evaluations of drinking and personality before and after treatment, and long-term follow-up procedures to be fully reported. It is hoped that this study will substantially decrease our ignorance about the effectiveness of LSD in alcoholism and that it will introduce a note of caution into the too rapid acceptance of unevaluated therapies. Finally, efforts will be made to examine the present status of LSD therapy in alcoholism and to suggest further areas for clinical investigation and experimentation.

EARLY USE OF LSD

Lysergic acid diethylamide (LSD) is a synthetic compound chemically related to a number of similar hallucinogenic drugs which occur naturally. Among these are mescaline in the peyote cactus, ololiuqui in morning glory seeds, bufotenine in mushrooms and toadstools, and harmine in vines. The most important of these for understanding the psychiatric uses of LSD is peyote as none of the others has had extensive or long use. It has been suggested by certain ethnographers (Slotkin, 1956) that frequent use of peyote has cured alcoholics. This belief has been assimilated into the LSD literature (e.g., Cohen, 1964, p. 21) and the first clinical trials of LSD in alcoholism seem (Unger, 1963) to have been based on this expectation. Consequently, the proposition demands careful appraisal.

The use of peyote among North American Indians has had a long and stormy history. Widespread use of peyote probably began in the early 1800's in northern Mexico (LaBarre, 1964) although documentary information on peyote in Mexico dates from the sixteenth century. During this early period it was used as a fetish in battle and to heal wounds. Ritual usage began in the early 1800's among the Apaches, Comanches, Kiowas, and other Plains Indians. During this period elaborate rituals were constructed for the gathering and consumption of peyote buttons. It was customarily eaten by peyotists sitting in a group around a specially constructed altar. Special prayers, bible readings, and ritual actions were necessary before peyote could be eaten, and, indeed, a formal religion eventually developed around the use of peyote among the Plains and other Indian peoples. Today its main features seem to involve frequent practice of the peyote rite and a belief in the power of peyote to cure illness, and to deliver knowledge, understanding, and tranquility, as well as the acceptance of certain ethical principles. This ethical system is a humanitarian and family-centered one which emphasizes brotherly love, care of the family, economic self-reliance, and the avoidance of alcohol. Indeed, there are numerous early and modern ethnographic references to the incompatibility of peyote and alcohol (Slotkin, 1956; LaBarre, 1964) and an important part of the modern peyote ethic is the total avoidance of alcohol, especially during and prior to the ritual. In Mexico, however, peyote was commonly drunk with alcoholic drinks and hence the antagonism between the two is not wholly physiological.

Historically, peyotism was part of a southwestern Indian cure for alcoholism. LaBarre (1964) has stated that "many Navajos have become peyotists for the express purpose of solving their drinking problems"; however, he doubts that peyotism really does cure alcoholism and cites several cases of acute alcoholism among ardent peyotists. He has also observed drinking among peyotists. Slotkin, however, quotes early first-hand reports to the contrary: "many members I have known twenty-five or thirty years, who formerly had been greatly addicted to the use of liquors and tobacco, and other vices; all have quit these bad habits and live for their religion" (p. 112); and "it cures us of our temporal ills, as well as those of a spiritual nature. It takes away the desire for strong drink. I, myself, have been cured of a loathsome disease, too horrible to mention. So have hundreds of others. Hundreds of confirmed drunkards have been dragged from their downward way" (p. 140).

In conclusion, it appears that close involvement in the peyote religion was probably responsible for arresting or curing alcoholic drinking although some failures have also been noted. However, any alleviation of drinking that occurred in this way could be attributable to membership in a group with a strong anti-alcohol ideology and the social support that it entails, rather than to a specific peyote–alcohol antagonism.

5

It is clear that peyote has a much longer history of use than do the lysergic acid compounds. LaBarre (1964) found evidence that peyote and mescal were used in Pre-Columbian Mexico, or at least 470 years ago. Lysergic acid as a hallucinogenic has had a much shorter history. By now, it is probably well known that Hofmann accidently discovered the hallucinogenic properties of LSD in 1943, although he appears to have taken little interest in its therapeutic properties at the time. Stoll (1947) repeated Hofmann's studies and began the first administration of the drug to mentally ill patients. He experimented informally with LSD and reports circulated that it had provoked a suicide in one of his patients. Surprisingly, Stoll never specifically reported on this suicide and it may well be apocryphal. Nevertheless early anxiety about such matters (e.g., Unger, 1963) seems to have retarded the therapeutic use of the drug.

The possibility that LSD could create a special awareness or insights valuable in therapy was not immediately realized. At first LSD was considered to be a psychotomimetic drug producing experiences and behavior similar to those found in psychoses. It was widely reported that the LSD experience allowed the study and understanding of schizophrenic psychoses in an experimental fashion. For example, psychiatrists spoke of "experimental schizo-phrenia-like symptoms" (Rinkel *et al.*, 1952) or of "model psy-choses induced by LSD-25" (Bercel *et al.*, 1956). Actually, many of the subjective reactions to LSD suggest schizophrenic symp-toms, although there are wide variations in the number and severity of the possible schizoid responses to LSD.

Typically, normal individuals after about 100 μg of LSD report visual illusions and hallucinations, disturbed time senses and body concepts, and feelings of depersonalization and unreality; they demonstrate poverty and looseness of thought, inattention, and impaired judgment and concentration. Observations made of persons given LSD usually also show "schizoid-type" distur-bances in language, blunting of affect, suspiciousness, underactivity, lack of spontaneity, and in some cases stupor and catatonia. In addition, psychological test results obtained during LSD sessions demonstrate abnormalities clearly similar to schizophrenic or paranoid states (Bercel *et al.*, 1956). While these subjective reports and observations suggest the more florid outbursts of schizophrenic patients, they do not constitute the whole LSD experience for all persons. There are many responses to LSD which are not typically schizophrenic. One general set of such responses is physiological and comprises giddiness, fainting, tremor, shaking, occasional abdominal cramps, physical weakness, sweating, and shivering (Linton and Langs, 1962; Rinkel *et al.*, 1952).

It has also been reported that the LSD reaction lacks many of the the typical features of schizophrenia. For example, major delusions, or ideas of grandeur or persecution are rarely seen in normals given LSD. Also, auditory hallucinations, clouding of consciousness, memory loss, and profound intellectual disorganization are relatively rare responses to LSD (Linton and Langs, 1962; Rinkel, *et al.*, 1952), but common in natural schizophrenic disorders. It appears, at present, that LSD does not create a clear analogue of the usual schizophrenic reaction or even the acute schizophrenic states.

A major part of the interest in LSD stemmed from the possibility that some chemical substance such as LSD could actually be causing schizophrenia. There has been a recent change in thinking about such drugs and a shift in preference from "hallucinogenic" to "psychedelic" or "mind-manifesting" as terms establishing their effects. LSD itself does not occur naturally in the body, but substances with properties similar to it have been identified. Several naturally occurring derivations of adrenaline—adrenochrome and adrenolutin—are also hallucinogens (Osmond and Smythies, 1952). LSD greatly increases adrenochrome levels in the blood and this increase may be part of the mechanism of hallucinogenic action for LSD. It has been argued then that schizophrenia is caused by some hallucinogen similar to LSD, such as adrenolutin or adrenochrome (Osmond and Smythies, 1952; Hoffer, Osmond, and Smythies, 1954). Many early studies of LSD were concerned with this biochemical theory of schizophrenia. However, a number of difficulties have developed around the lack of similarity between the LSD experience and schizophrenia, and around the exact relation of adrenochrome to schizophrenia. This phase of the work with LSD has had at least a temporary eclipse, and far more current interest exists in the use of LSD as a therapeutic agent, and in comparing its benefits with its possible dangers.

DANGERS OF LSD

It has long been recognized that certain dangerous complications can arise from the use of LSD as an investigatory or therapeutic drug. Usually, it is claimed that the actual dangers from LSD administration are slight (Smith, 1964; Cohen and Ditman, 1962) and probably not more serious than those attached to many other effective drugs, deaths having been reported from therapy with many antibiotics (e.g., penicillin and chloromycetin) and with simple analgesics such as aspirin and codeine. In the main, the possible undesirable effects of LSD may be suicide, homicide, addiction, and the creation or uncovering of psychotic states in the user. The actual number of patients showing one or more of these complications is apparently small, but this number may be greatly underreported.

Although every drug is probably fatally toxic at very high doses, LSD has a relatively low toxicity. There have been no deaths reported in man due to its toxic effects and the lethal dose for humans is not known. Amounts 15 times as high as those necessary to produce an LSD reaction (100 μg) have been taken without permanent ill effects. Bunnell (1966) has estimated from various studies of lethality in non-human animals that the lethal dose of LSD is about 14 mg/kg. This, of course, is far beyond the dose being given in experimental or therapeutic situations.

Considerable concern has been expressed over the possibility that LSD leads to suicide in some of its users. Hoffer (cited in Smith, 1964) has reviewed the results of studies using a total of 5000 subjects in various experimental and therapeutic studies. This review yielded only five cases of suicide subsequent to LSD use; four of these occurred some time after LSD had been discontinued and hence in these cases the direct association with the LSD experience can be questioned. Nevertheless, LSD has been found to have prolonged and profound psychological effects in some persons and the possibilities of related suicides cannot be easily dismissed. Only two of these suicides were considered by Cohen (Abramson, 1960, p. 227) to be directly attributable to the LSD experience. These have been tentatively related to a "sudden upsurge of overwhelming and guilt-loaded material which the patient cannot incorporate, and the therapist fails to provide the necessary support." The investigators reporting these suicides (Abramson, 1960) have not directly attributed them to LSD but rather to long-term psychiatric problems, chiefly depression. Of course, the small number of actual suicides reported makes the LSD-suicide relationship difficult to establish with certainty.

All of the suicides reported occurred during therapeutic rather than experimental trials. The experimental studies, of course, would contain larger groups of normal persons than would the therapeutic studies and hence one would expect fewer suicides among them, both in general and in response to LSD. It might also be noted in passing that the numerous reports on the use of peyote by Plains Indians contain no mention of associated suicide. Suicide risks should be substantially reduced where LSD patients are carefully screened for psychiatric problems and where long-term follow-ups or hospitalization after LSD are employed.

One difficulty in accepting the reported incidence of LSD-related suicides concerns the procedures followed during many LSD studies. Many of them have used *very* short follow-up periods or none at all. For example, studies of LSD therapy with alcoholics (Smart and Storm, 1964) report follow-up periods varying from two months to three years and similarly wide variations can be found in studies with other types of patients. Some therapeutic studies have been reported which involved no follow-up beyond the LSD experience (Chandler and Hartman, 1960). In addition, it is clear that routine follow-up procedures are not common in studies investigating the basic psychological or physiological properties of LSD in a non-therapeutic setting (e.g., Linton and Langs, 1962). All of these considerations raise questions about the validity of present estimates of the number of LSD-related suicides. The incidence of 5 cases in 5000 appears to be very low, but this may be a gross underreporting of the true incidence; there is little to help us judge its validity at present.

If there is some uncertainty about the suicide hazard in the carefully controlled use of LSD, there is even more uncertainty in its uncontrolled non-medical use. There have been many reports of black-market sales of hallucinogenic drugs (Cohen and Ditman, 1963) and of their use by non-medical personnel on university campuses, in coffee houses and in other unprotected settings (LaBarre, 1964; Cohen, 1966; Subcommittee on Narcotics Addiction, 1966). Indeed, some of these "reports" were apparently responsible for the introduction of strict legal control over such drugs in Canada and the United States. An important point here is that almost nothing is known about the suicide rate in the non-medical use of LSD and reliable methods for gathering this type of information are not available. Presumably, some hazard attaches to non-medical use but we have little information in the way of a systematic study—only isolated case reports (e.g., LaBarre, 1964).

A number of investigators have mentioned that LSD leads to great emotionality and aggressive behavior; the possibility that homicide can result should also be mentioned. The only definite case of homicide following LSD was reported by Knudsen (1964). In this instance a 25-year-old woman murdered her boy friend two days after the last of five LSD sessions. The murder was not, of course, committed during the acute effects of LSD but a close connection is apparent, as the desire to murder the boy friend was expressed during at least one LSD session. In this patient LSD appeared to release aggressive drives and to weaken self-control. The diagnosis was psychopathic personality with chronic alcoholism, so that more complicated factors than a simple drug effect were operating. One additional homicide may have been committed by an LSD user (MacLeod, 1966), although the connection between the LSD experience and the homicide is uncertain. A medical school dropout, reported to have taken LSD frequently, is alleged to have murdered his mother-in-law, but this case has not been clarified as yet. Observers reported that he had been wandering aimlessly in an apparently drugged state some hours before the murder.

10

Addiction has also been mentioned as a possible complicating factor in the use of LSD. The drug has been shown to produce important and striking personality changes and perhaps any drug with these features has at least some addictive liability. Addiction can be understood in the pharmacological sense of a physical dependence marked by increased tolerance and specific withdrawal symptoms on termination of a drug's use. But addiction can also be understood in the psychological sense of dependence on a drug to preserve psychological functioning, or as drug use sufficient to produce some psychological or social damage (e.g., to employability, family relationships, personality functioning, moral and ethical controls). It is frequently found that volunteers for LSD do not wish to take the drug again—particularly if it is not given as a therapeutic agent. Consequently, few have the chance to develop tolerance to it, although tolerance can be rapidly created with frequent use (Bunnell, 1966). There are numerous reports of long series of LSD administrations (e.g., 200 to 300 occasions, see Cohen and Ditman, 1963) but no cases of pharmacological addiction indicated by physical withdrawal symptoms. Also, the literature on the peyote cult among American Indians describes no case of peyote addiction. In fact, the non-addictive nature of peyote became an argument for maintaining its freedom from legal control (Slotkin, 1956). Cohen and Ditman (1963) reported a case in which a woman took LSD 200 to 300 times in a one-year period and hence seemed to have developed a psychological dependence on it, but no withdrawal signs were noted. Unfortunately, the pharmacological effects of long-term LSD administration have not been explored experimentally. It may be that its low addictive liability is mainly a function of the small number of sessions usually given.

Little has been said, so far, about the possibility that LSD can result in long-term complications of a psychotic or depressive nature—without suicide. Again, there are few complications when the drug is given to "normal" subjects in the course of experimentation and most complications appear during therapeutic or non-medical use. The actual number of such complications is unknown at present but most of them appeared in pre-psychotic

11

persons or in those with a family history of psychosis. Cohen and Ditman (1962) reviewed LSD complications up to 1960 and found that the rate of psychoses in LSD therapy was 0.18 per cent. There is very little knowledge about the psychotic complications resulting from non-medical use, although several cases have been reported by Cohen and Ditman (1963). Once again, the true rate may be quite different from that reported.

Detailed information on psychotic complications has been collected only for medically supervised experimental and therapeutic trials. However, there are a number of isolated reports of complications from unsupervised use. For example, during 10 months in 1965 the Bellevue Hospital in New York had 52 cases of prolonged psychoses resulting from LSD (Subcommittee on Narcotics Addiction, 1966). All of the affected persons had taken LSD in unsupervised settings and in unknown doses. The predominant manifestations were overwhelming fear (12 cases), violent uncontrolled urges (9 cases) including two homicide attempts, and visual hallucinations (15 cases). Twelve of the 52 affected cases had had previous psychotic episodes or prior psychiatric treatment. Most of those seen at Bellevue recovered within 48 hours (30 cases), but 6 had prolonged psychoses requiring hospitalization in psychiatric institutions. Similar findings were reported by Cohen (1966) who studied 40 cases of prolonged LSD psychoses admitted to the Los Angeles County Hospital in a single month. Ditman (1966) also reported on 73 cases of LSD psychoses seen by psychiatrists in the Los Angeles area. Again it appeared that the taking of LSD in unsupervised settings is attractive to emotionally unstable persons since half had had psychotherapy before or during the LSD experience. The following conditions were found to predispose LSD users to prolonged psychotic experiences: (1) repeated ingestion; (2) emotional instability in the user; (3) concurrent addiction to other drugs (e.g., alcohol, amphetamines); (4) ingestion without knowledge of the taker; (5) non-medical controls or administration; (6) doses over 600 μg; (7) concurrent use with other drugs (e.g., alcohol, barbiturates, amphetamines). As would be expected, it is not known what proportion of unsupervised LSD experiences result in psychoses. However, the impression gained is that this is the most dangerous way in which LSD may be taken, partly because it seems attractive to those with existing psychiatric problems.

One further difficulty with LSD is that there are suspicions that it can create the same complications in the therapist as in the patient. This has been commented upon by Cohen especially (Cohen, 1964) but suggested by others (LaBarre, 1964). Cohen briefly described several cases of "therapist breakdown" involving psychotic illness, marked depressions, suicide, and "megalomaniacal ideas of grandeur." Unfortunately, none of these cases is reported in detail, although Cohen described the case of a secretary, employed by an LSD practitioner, who took many doses and developed long-standing panic states, hallucinations, and depressions. Perhaps a similar instance of therapist involvement can be found in the Alpert-Leary case at Harvard University. In 1961 Dr. Richard Alpert and Dr. Timothy Leary, teachers at Harvard University, began studies of the use of psilocybin in rehabilitating prisoners. They soon began giving hallucinogens in cocktail party settings, administering them to undergraduates and graduates indiscriminately, and taking hallucinogens themselves at the same time as they were to record and observe LSD reactions in others. The scientific standards of their work with LSD suffered markedly, received much criticism, and eventually led to their dismissal from Harvard in 1963. They then set up a series of "Freedom Centers" (under the International Federation for Internal Freedom) in which "experiments" with hallucinogens and "multiple family living" are conducted. Both Alpert and Leary reported taking LSD on numerous occasions and perhaps their changed attitudes toward research and evaluation and their wholehearted devotion to hallucinogens[1] represent a type of risk to which LSD practitioners are prone. Cohen (1964) has stated that many such practitioners themselves, take LSD to excess, but he gives no clear instance of ensuing harmful effects.

[1]At one time Leary argued that hallucinogens should be considered as vitamins which we lacked and that they should be made as readily available as other foods.

2. Use of LSD in Psychiatric Treatment

DESPITE THE POSSIBLE DANGERS associated with LSD it has been extensively used in various types of psychiatric therapy. Investigations of its acute effects and of its therapeutic potential with schizophrenics and neurotics have largely predated its use with alcoholics.

The first report of the use of LSD in psychotherapy appeared in 1950 (Busch and Johnson, 1950). Nine years later, a conference held on LSD in psychotherapy included participants who, collectively, had treated more than 1000 adult patients with this drug (Abramson, 1960). In 1964 a bibliography of the literature on the use of LSD in psychotherapy, based on English-language publications alone, contained 60 items (Unger, 1964). The total number of psychiatric patients treated with LSD is at least several thousand. The number of normal volunteers or psychiatric patients given LSD in experimental rather than treatment settings equals or exceeds the number given it for therapeutic reasons. There is, then, a large body of experience with the drug and with its effects on human subjects. In spite of this, the evidence that LSD is effective with any particular type of patient, or in any particular therapeutic setting, is not conclusive. The specific acute effects of the drug under various conditions are inadequately known in any systematic way, and, further, the mechanisms of drug action are not fully understood.

There are many reasons for this state of affairs. At the time of Unger's (1964) bibliography, "not a single methodologically-acceptable controlled study of the efficacy of LSD-assisted psychotherapy" had been performed. As Unger points out, such studies are very rare with any type of psychotherapy. It would seem, however, that there is rather less excuse for the failure to include certain controls in the case of LSD than in psychotherapy generally. The majority of therapists use it as an addition to their normal therapeutic procedures. It would be a simple matter to determine on a random basis which patients were to receive this addition and to compare the outcome of treatment in these patients to the outcome in those not receiving the drug. Random assignment to treatment conditions is the essential element in a controlled study, and the fact that patients given a new treatment had not *yet* responded to other forms of treatment (the control in most reports) is not an adequate substitute. Furthermore, the involvement of LSD in the treatment process is discrete and relatively brief—in some studies, a single session—so that the problem of defining and controlling the beginning and the end of treatment, or of this special aspect of a larger treatment process, is relatively simple compared with that in the conventional forms of psychotherapy.

It must be admitted, however, that even if such a procedure had been used much more frequently than is the case, the situation would be only partially clarified. There are many specific assumptions about the psychological effects of LSD which mediate its therapeutic effectiveness and many generalizations about the dependence of these effects on the setting and the personality of the patient which need to be tested apart from the over-all effectiveness of psychotherapy which includes LSD.

Lindemann and Von Felsinger (1961) have pointed out the complexities involved in evaluating the psychological effects of any drug. They distinguish drug-specific from personality-specific effects, primary effects from secondary elaboration or adaptations to the primary effects, and the interaction of these with the psychosocial setting, including the expectations of the subject and his relations to others while he is under the influence of the drug. Nowlis and Nowlis (1956) and Schachter (1965), among others, have demonstrated experimentally the importance of social psychological variables in the psychological effects of drugs other than LSD.

The importance of the total setting is not only recognized, but is emphasized by those who use LSD therapeutically. According to Savage *et al.* (1965), unless the experiences produced by LSD "occur in a secure setting, with sufficient emotional support where S feels safe to encounter the bizarre and often powerful manifestations of his own mind unharassed by tests, interpretations, and the coldly precise scientific or analytic attitudes, the only result can be confusion and paranoia." Many experimental studies, of course, have exposed subjects under LSD to "harassment" by tests, and in many treatment settings, interpretation is a prominent part of the patient–therapist interaction under LSD (see, e.g., Abramson, 1960); nevertheless, the emphasis on psychosocial factors is there. Similarly, Hartman points out that in his group of investigators, the Jungians "will get the transcendental experience in the patient much faster" than the Freudians, whereas the latter "will evoke the patient's childhood memories much more quickly than the two Jungians in the group" (Abramson, 1960, p. 132). A complete evaluation of LSD in treatment would have to include the investigations of these and similar claims; it would have to compare outcomes of treatment in various settings; and, in any particular setting, it would have to compare outcomes with LSD and without, while the rest of the procedure was held constant.

In this chapter we will review and attempt to evaluate, tentatively, the evidence for the effectiveness of LSD in the treatment of psychiatric patients, largely psychoneurotics and those with character disorders. We will also review the neurophysiological and psychological effects of LSD as reported from clinical observations and from experimental studies with human and animal subjects. In this way a frame of reference within which the results of treatment can be viewed may be established. This will be followed by a more detailed account of selected treatment studies representative of the range of therapeutic uses of LSD and an evaluation of its current status in the context of psychotherapy.

PSYCHOLOGICAL AND NEUROPHYSIOLOGICAL EFFECTS

In most of the studies cited in this section LSD has been administered in doses of 75 to 150 μg. The dosage used in treatment may be much higher. More usually it is at the upper end of this range.

Neurophysiological

No effort will be made here to review all of the studies relevant to the non-neural biochemical effects of LSD since this has been adequately done by Hoffer (1965) and by Bunnell (1966). Our concern is with the effects of LSD at several different neurophysiological levels—those of synaptic transmission, nerve tracts and pathways both discrete and diffuse, and the more global levels affected by gross surgical ablation.

At the biochemical level, Freedman (1963) has shown that LSD effects relate to the levels of the brain amines, especially serotonin and noradrenaline. Pre-treatment with reserpine increases the behavioral effects of LSD in rats during the period of reserpine-induced, lowered serotonin levels. LSD administration quickly results in increased serotonin and decreased noradrenaline levels in the rat brain. Prolonged stress in the rat, for example, a prolonged cold swim, has a similar effect. It appears that LSD produces an effect on brain amines which mimics vigorous exercise. Resnick (1964, 1965) found that in normal human subjects reserpine enhances and mono-amine oxidase inhibitors attenuate LSD effects, thus paralleling the rat experiments.

At the synaptic level, Purpura (1956) has hypothesized that LSD depresses axodendritic transmission and enhances axosomatic transmission. This hypothesis is compatible with his findings of increased discrete sensory pathway transmission to the primary sensory cortex, coupled with reduced transmission through the diffuse sensory system and from the primary sensory to the association cortex. In the former axosomatic transmission is present, and in the latter two axodendritic transmission prevails.

A current argument in the literature concerns the effects of LSD on sensory transmission. Does LSD decrease or increase filtration of sensory input? The pertinent work on this subject has been summarized by Key (1965a). It appears that a meaningful study of LSD effects requires unanesthetized animals, with chronically implanted subcortical electrodes, which are tested in rigidly controlled environmental situations. Key indicates that in the unanesthetized animal LSD overcomes the effects of habituation, resulting in increased attention to previously irrelevant stimuli.

LSD activates the diffuse reticular substance producing behavioral arousal and EEG neocortical desynchronization (Key, 1965b). Hippocampal cortical discharges are synchronized, producing abnormal theta trains in cats. Thus neocortical effects contrast strikingly with paleocortical effects. Centrally induced hippocampal seizures are prolonged (Killam and Killam, 1956) in keeping with the notion of hypersynchrony of the old cortex.

Cerebral ablation experiments by Baldwin, Lewis, and Bach (1959), using monkeys, show that LSD behavioral effects require intact temporal lobes. Bilateral frontal lobectomy, or bilateral *medial* temporal lobectomy did not modify the behavioral effect of LSD in monkeys. Bilateral ablation of the lateral halves of both temporal lobes, however, did abolish the LSD-behavioral effect.

In experiments involving classical Pavlovian conditioning of animals, LSD has been shown by computer analysis to bring back electrophysiological correlates of extinction in the hippocampus and to modify the correlates of "discrimination" for a period of up to a week following the LSD injection (Sheatz and Bogdanski, 1964). Wikler *et al.* (1965) have demonstrated that LSD creates pupil widening and reduces knee-jerk reflexes in human volunteers.

Monnier (1959) summarized the effects of LSD on physiological activity in animals as the following: sympathetic activation; activation of electroretinogram; inhibition of lateral geniculate at higher doses, and facilitation at lower ones; inhibition of occipitocortical potentials evoked by visual stimuli or electrical stimulation of the optic tracts; desynchronization of spontaneous cortical EEG activity; synchronization in the hippocampus; enhancement of cortical arousal response to sensory stimulation or to stimulation of the reticular formation; and inhibition of mediothalamic recruiting.

Behavioral

In comparison with placebo conditions, the performance of normal human subjects on objective tests is generally impaired or unaffected by LSD; performance is rarely enhanced. Two studies report decreased performance on standard intelligence tests (Levine *et al.*, 1955; Cohen, Fichman, and Eisner, 1958), and one, "little loss in efficiency" (Rinkel, 1958). Particular tests on which performance related to intelligence has been impaired include the following: digit span and other tests of memory (Jarvik, Abramson, and Hirsch, 1955; Kornetsky, Humphries, and Evarts, 1957; Silverstein and Klee, 1960), proverbs (Silverstein and Klee, 1958), the Porteus maze (Aronson and Klee, 1960), spatial relations (Abramson *et al.*, 1955), figure drawing (Silverstein and Klee, 1958), and arithmetic (Jarvik *et al.*, 1955). Performance on various psychomotor tasks has also been impaired, among them dual pursuit rotor learning (Silverstein and Klee, 1960) and mirror drawing (Orsini and Benda, 1960). Impairment of these tasks is generally attributed to difficulties in concentrating under LSD and increased concreteness in tasks requiring abstraction.

On measures involving fluency of response and reaction time, the former is decreased under experimental conditions, and the latter increased. Verbal reaction time is also increased (Abramson, Jarvik, and Hirsch, 1955; Weintraub, Silverstein, and Klee, 1959), while productivity on the Rorschach is decreased (Stoll, 1952; Rinkel, 1956). LSD, compared with epinephrine, decreased the intelligibility of speech samples studied with Cloze analysis (Honigfeld, 1964). This study, and the Rorschach and association studies cited, provide evidence that the frequency of unusual or improbable responses is increased under LSD.

LSD also appears to increase perceptual field dependence, or the interfering effects of misleading contexts on visual perception. Effects of this type were shown with the rod-and-frame test (Liebert, Wapner, and Werner, 1957), with the Heiss-Sandler figure test (Krus and Wapner, 1959), and with the Stroop color-word test (Wapner and Krus, 1960).

Changes in perception demonstrated in objective tests include raised visual threshold (Carlson, 1958), and changes in size constancy (Weckowicz, 1959) and body image (Liebert, Werner, and Wapner, 1958). In tests of color perception, Hartman and Hollister (1963) found decreased hue discrimination, but enhanced color phenomena to normally inadequate stimuli. Under stabilized image conditions, a target stimulus pattern was less subject to fading and reappeared more often under LSD. There were also more reported distortions of the target stimulus under the drug (Kohn and Bryden, 1965). Several studies have found changes in time judgment (Boardman, Goldstone, and Lhamon, 1957; Benda and Orsini, 1959; Aronson, Silverstein, and Klee, 1959).

Animal studies show decreased or highly erratic response rates for positive reinforcers (Blough, 1957; Malis, Brodie, and Moreno 1960; Ray and Marrazzi, 1960; Stein, 1960). The only instances of decreased latency of responding involved the unconditioned response to an aversive stimulus and a conditioned avoidance response (Taeschler, Weidman, and Cerletti, 1960).

Subjective Psychological Effects

One of the most complete and careful studies of the subjective effects of LSD was performed by Linton and Langs (1962). Since their findings are in general agreement with other studies of normal volunteers under LSD, it will be summarized in some detail.

This study employed a 74-item questionnaire. Items were selected on the basis of reports in the literature on the subjective effects of LSD and on the basis of psychoanalytic hypotheses. The questionnaire was administered on the day before the experimental day, several times during the experimental day, and on the following day. The subjects were male professional actors, paid volunteers ranging in age from 21 to 42 with a median age of 28. Only those volunteers judged on the basis of clinical information to have psychotic or paranoid tendencies were excluded from participation. Thirty subjects received 100 μg of LSD on the experimental day; twenty received a placebo. All subjects went through the same extensive testing procedure. On the experimental day this involved almost continuous testing from 8:30 A.M. until 5:00 P.M.

Those items which were checked by more than two-thirds of the LSD subjects at some time during the experimental day and which also differentiated significantly between LSD and placebo

20

subjects included difficulty in concentration, impaired judgment, difficulty in retaining ideas, and disturbances in body image and time sense. Changes in mood were frequent but the type of mood change was variable. Physical effects and changes in body image had the earliest onset under LSD and were frequently accompanied by fears of loss of control. Mood changes tended to occur next, and difficulties in thinking and concentration followed. Reports that the meanings of stimuli and events in the environment had altered, or that they had lost their meaning, came later and occurred in between 50 and 60 per cent of the LSD subjects. Childhood memories and "transcendental" feelings of unity and deep insight, both of which are stressed in the therapeutic usefulness of LSD, were relatively rare, although items with related content were checked more frequently than in the placebo group. In therapeutic settings, of course, deliberate attempts are made to facilitate such experience, or such interpretations of more primary LSD reactions. This was not done in the Linton and Langs study, and subjects were kept occupied with testing during the drug day.

The questionnaire items were grouped on the basis of similarity of content into 17 *a priori* scales. In a later report, Linton and Langs (1964) present the results of a factor analysis of the intercorrelations among these *a priori* scales. Four empirical scales emerge from this analysis—two of these are interpreted as extreme versions of the other two, with which they are correlated. These presumably more typical patterns appear to differ essentially in the direction of the predominant affective reaction. The first combines feelings of improved functioning, capacity to perceive new meanings, and elation. Behaviorally, subjects high in this pattern were judged to be more confused, more verbal and open, and sillier under LSD. The second pattern was characterized by alterations in body image and a generalized inhibitory effect indicated in perceived slowing of thought and movement. Behaviorally subjects high in this pattern were judged to be more anxious, to show more bodily concern, and to be more passive. Subjects with the less frequent pattern correlated with the first, euphoric pattern showed paranoid tendencies; those with the rarer pattern correlated with the more introverted pattern showed marked overt anxiety, and expressed fears of losing their mind.

Changes similar to those described by Linton and Langs' subjects and similar variations from subject to subject are reported elsewhere with persons given LSD for research purposes. However, the less controlled the study, the less standard and objective the measures, and the more clinical the setting, the more extreme are the reactions reported.

One interesting study suggests the importance of the setting in determining whether the affective reaction to LSD is predominantly expansive and positive, or predominantly negative (Slater, Morimoto, and Hyde, 1957). Seventy-two normal subjects received LSD in groups of two or more, or alone. Those given LSD in groups tended to have manic reactions and to show elation. Those given LSD alone showed more thought and speech disturbance, anxiety, depression, underactivity, somatic symptoms, sensory illusions, and hallucinations. Subjects studied under individual and group conditions did not differ in incidence of body image disturbances or impairment of attention.

Ditman and Whittlesey (1959) used 300 cards, each with a statement potentially relevant to the LSD experience. Subjects (including psychiatric patients) selected those ten or fewer which were most descriptive of their own experience. Euphoria, a sense of wonderment, perceptual distortion, increased alertness, somatic discomfort, and increased rate of thought were items characterizing the LSD experience. Dissociation of thought, inappropriate affect, catatonic features, depersonalization, and hostility were common LSD reactions of 100 normal volunteers in studies conducted by Rinkel (1958). Hallucinations were rare, as they appear to be in most reports. Autonomic changes preceded the psychological effects. Isbell (1959) found the LSD experience to be characterized by feelings of strangeness, difficulty in thinking, anxiety, altered perception, hallucinations, and altered body image, compared with reports and behavior of the same (normal) subjects under placebo. Autonomic changes also occurred. Manic changes, including feelings of elation and euphoria, were common in a study by Lebovits, Visotsky, and Ostfeld (1960), although despondency and anxiety also occurred under LSD. Feelings of depersonalization and disturbances in body image were reported. Alterations in visual perception were also found.

Abramson *et al.* (1955) reported a correlation of the occurrence of psychotic symptoms (hallucinations and delusions) and perceptual distortions with dose level over a range of 0 to 225 μg. There was no such correlation with anxiety under LSD.

PROPOSED MECHANISMS OF ACTION

With LSD it is too early to specify the chain of events leading from the biochemical to the behavioral level. It is possible, however, to formulate some hypotheses about the basic effects of LSD which account for the variety, and the variability, of specific behavioral effects reported. Three basic effects, not necessarily independent physiologically, may be assumed. These are general arousal, alteration in sensory input to the cortex, and alteration in the relative strengths of learned responses and associations. The ways in which these hypothetical effects could account for most of the specific changes found under LSD will be elaborated below.

The most consistent and immediate effect of LSD appears to be sympathetic activation. The less consistent reports of EEG arousal in the neocortex may indicate that the autonomic changes are a part of a general arousal reaction initiated by LSD. Schachter (1965) has shown that physiological arousal produced by drugs may or may not be accompanied by emotional experience and emotional behavior. Whether the subject experiences emotion depends upon his interpretation of the physiological changes which in turn depends upon what he has been led to expect. If he experiences emotion, the nature of the emotion will depend upon the cues in his immediate environment which have potential emotional significance and upon his interpretation of them. The subject's personality (his habitual response patterns) will also be an important determinant of the interpretation he places on his own physiological state and on the situation. Whatever the outcome, his overt behavior will tend to be congruent with his emotional state as he interprets it.

Many of the emotional and behavioral effects of LSD could be

23

accounted for on the basis of the activating effect of the drug, interpreted and elaborated by the subject. The activating effect makes it likely that some emotion will be experienced, except with very sophisticated subjects with highly investigative sets in familiar surroundings with familiar companions. What emotion is experienced, and what behavior ensues, should vary widely from person to person, and from situation to situation. In a group with others in the same circumstances, the heightened arousal might well be expressed in greater talkativeness and animation (for which the group setting provides a ready opportunity) and be interpreted (by the subject himself, as well as by others) as elation. In a strange setting, with unfamiliar people, where some nervousness may be already present, anxiety is perhaps more likely. When a subject is told, sometimes at great length, in advance of LSD, to expect to relive traumatic experiences from childhood, or to expect feelings of great insight and richness of experience, it is likely that he will be inclined to interpret a non-specific excitement in a manner consistent with those expectations. For obvious reasons, investigators seeking to clarify the effect of LSD avoid giving their subjects any specific expectations, and they find little consistency in emotional effects, except in finding some such effects. The therapist, using LSD in therapy, does prepare his patients as specifically as he can, and generally has strong convictions about the essential nature of the LSD experience which he attempts to convey.

The assumption that LSD results only in general arousal accounts for some of the findings reported, but not for all of them. It seems unlikely that *any* activating drug, in a dose producing an equivalent arousal effect, would produce the perceptual distortions consistently reported for LSD or the apparent abreactive effects often found in treatment settings. But the possibility should not be entirely ruled out that if suggestions were given with the proper thoroughness and conviction, and with the same aura that currently surrounds LSD, such effects might not be produced by another drug. It would be important in any test of this possibility that dosages of LSD and a control drug be adjusted to produce the same degree of general arousal.

There does seem to be evidence, however, for an effect of LSD in the primary sensory projection system. Those studies reporting an effect on the potentials recorded from the retina, and on transmission from the lateral geniculate in particular, suggest an alteration in sensory input. Such an effect would acount for the reports of frequent visual distortions after LSD. If this effect is not limited to the visual system, it would account also for the disturbances of body image and for the feelings of strangeness or unreality. These latter feelings, next to the autonomic effects, appear to be the most consistent and universal aspects of the drug experience. Once again, the subject will interpret and react to these changes, and his interpretation will reflect his expectations and the general setting.

A third possible mechanism which could account for LSD effects is an alteration in the relative strengths of learned responses and associations, resulting from a reduction in the strength of all learned patterns to a degree proportional to their original strength. The strength of dominant response patterns would be reduced more than the strength of weaker patterns. With random oscillation in momentary strength, the weaker patterns would be more likely to occur occasionally under drugged than under normal conditions. Stimulus support normally inadequate to elicit weaker responses, when the absolute differences between response strengths were greater, would more frequently elicit these responses under the drugged conditions. Such an effect might result from an alteration in cerebral metabolism or synaptic processes in the cortex, producing a kind of physiological "stimulus generalization decrement." A similar mechanism has been proposed to account for a lack of transfer of learned responses from drugged to non-drugged status (Overton, 1964; Otis, 1964), for loss of memory for events occurring during acute alcohol intoxication (Storm and Smart, 1965), and for the effects of electroconvulsive shock. This mechanism could account for the intellectual deterioration under LSD, for the greater concreteness and field dependence, and for the purportedly greater availability of personal (rather than conventional) associations and otherwise inaccessible memories. This interpretation has the advantage that it can account for the occasional persistence of some of the experiences under LSD and their repetition after the drug is no longer active. Altered perceptions, recovered memories, or unusual associations might be strengthened when they occur under the drug and have an increased probability of occurrence when the drug condition has disappeared.

These three basic effects in the total LSD experience would interact and reinforce each other. Arousal, beyond an optimal level, disorganizes behavior. Disturbances in visual and kinesthetic perception are frightening and raise the level of arousal. High arousal may raise some weak responses and remote associations above the response threshold. Unaccustomed difficulty in performing intellectual tasks, and the occurrence of unusual thoughts, may increase fear of loss of control. The reaction to all of these phenomena, however, would depend heavily on personality and social psychological variables. Unusual visual effects may be enjoyed, given appropriate expectations and a reassuring setting. Unusual associations may be interpreted as increased creativity and lead to elation rather than to anxiety. There is support for these interpretations in studies relating personality factors to a favorable or unfavorable attitude to the LSD experience (e.g., McGlothlin and Cohen, 1965).

The hypotheses put forward here are not radically different from the interpretations of the LSD experience offered by those who are enthusiastic about the therapeutic potential of the drug, whether their approach to its use is psychoanalytic in orientation or is based on a transcendental, quasi-religious interpretation of LSD and its beneficial effects. These writers (e.g., Smith, 1959; Chwelos, *et al.*, 1959) also emphasize the importance of social-psychological factors in determining the emotional quality of the experience, their accounts differing from the present one in their use of romantic and picturesque descriptions of what occurs under LSD. They differ more basically, however, in their belief that what occurs under LSD in the conditions they regard as optimal is in some way more "real," "true," or "fundamental" than the experiences most people have without the drug. We, on the other hand, would regard the psychological state produced by the drug as one in which persons in general, and some persons more than others, are peculiarly susceptible to concerted attempts at social influence. We would expect that the more subjective and attitudinal the criteria for change, and the less specific and behavioral, the more change would be found; that the more convinced the therapist is of the value of LSD, the more radical the acute effect of the drug on the subject or patient would be and the greater the claims of lasting benefit by the patient.

TREATMENT OF NEUROTICS AND SCHIZOPHRENICS

There are two major types of approach to the use of LSD in psychotherapy for neuroses and personality disorders. In the first, the drug is used as an adjunct to conventional, usually psycho-analytic, methods of psychotherapy. The psychological effects of the drug, together with appropriate preparation of the patient and an appropriate setting, are considered to facilitate the attain-ment of therapeutic goals, that is, the release of unconscious material, the reliving of traumatic experiences, and the analysis of transference, all of which are then utilized in further therapeutic sessions with or without LSD. The other approach regards the LSD experience as therapeutic in itself, if it is approached by the patient in the proper way and accepted rather than resisted. The relationship between therapist and patient is used as an aid to the LSD experience, the effect of which is said to be a temporary expansion of consciousness. It induces changes in the patient's value and belief system, and associated changes in behavior, in the direction of self-actualization (Savage, et al., 1965).

There is a great deal of variation from therapist to therapist in the procedural details of LSD treatment, regardless of the general approach. Most often, therapists using LSD as an aid to therapy employ the drug in repeated sessions, beginning with a small dose and increasing it in successive sessions until a satisfactory level of response is reached, usually at a dose of about 150 μg. Those who regard the "psychedelic" experience as primary typically employ a single, large dose of 200–300 μg, and sometimes a much larger one, depending on the patient's response. This variation in pro-cedure makes it difficult and perhaps unreasonable to expect to evaluate "LSD treatment" as a single entity. If these variations are important, however, we might expect concomitant variation in outcomes, particularly in view of claims that failure to meet specified conditions may have antitherapeutic results (Savage and Stolaroff, 1965).

Smart and Storm (1964) have summarized the requirements for research into the efficacy of any new treatment. These include the use of a control group receiving no treatment or another form of treatment against which the new treatment can be evaluated. There should be random assignment to any groups to be compared. Some objective measures, or subjective ratings uncontaminated by knowledge of the treatment the patient received, are required to assess outcomes. These assessments should be made before and after treatment, so that change can be detected. Post-treatment measures should be obtained at relatively fixed intervals after treatment to assess the persistence of therapeutic change. To determine whether the effects of a drug are attributable to its pharmacologic properties, a control group receiving a placebo or relatively inert drug must be employed. If placebos are used, the study should be double-blind, that is, neither the treatment personnel nor the patient should know which drug the latter receives.

No report of treatment results with LSD encountered in the literature meets all of these requirements. Many meet none of them. Outcome is often assessed by the unsupported claims of patients or the equally unsupported claims of the therapist, both with full knowledge of the treatment received. Subjects for LSD treatment are sometimes self-selected, but usually they are therapist-selected on the basis of varying and largely subjective criteria. Under these conditions, it is impossible to arrive at firm conclusions. It is, however, possible to arrive at a notion of the general level of results claimed, and to compare this with estimates of outcome from other methods of psychotherapy.

The reports summarized below are concerned with the effects of one form or another of treatment with LSD in non-psychotic adult psychiatric patients. Reports of psychotic patients treated with this drug are rare in the literature. In withdrawn, chronic, or catatonic states, LSD may re-activate acute symptoms, and may produce greater access. This effect is found in the report by Bender, Faretra, and Cobrini (1963) on their use of the drug with psychotic children. No other therapeutic claims for LSD in psychotics were encountered, and no studies of substantial numbers of adult psychotics systematically given LSD for therapeutic purposes have been found. (Reports of treatment of alcoholics with LSD are omitted, as they will be reviewed in the next chapter.)

Baker (1964) reported on a series of 150 patients with non-psychotic functional disorders who were given from 25 to 2000 μg of LSD per session for from one to ten sessions. These were clinical trials with no systematic assessment before or after treatment. It was the author's impression that two-thirds of the patients benefited from the LSD procedure, but no other supporting evidence is given. The model for treatment was psychoanalytic. The author emphasizes the increased capacity to "perceptualize the transference" under LSD. Preparation of the patient and the setting were designed to maximize this effect. Both doctor and nurse, prepared to play the roles of parental surrogates, were present. A single, massive dose of LSD was given in Baker's study although a "small-dose method" is described. This contrasts with the procedure more usually employed by psychoanalysts, one involving smaller doses and repeated sessions on the assumption that small doses are better. This assumption is based on the dangers of "overwhelming the ego" with a too massive and too rapid return of repressed material. In this connection, Baker's report that four patients became psychotic and required electro-convulsive therapy may be relevant. However, "none were permanently harmed," and the over-all incidence of improvement, judged by the only criterion provided, is comparable with other reports using quite different procedures. Another aspect of Baker's treatment procedure which contrasts with others, particularly with those recommended by adherents of the psychedelic approach, is the routine use of restraint. Baker proposes a number of indications and contraindications for LSD treatment, but no empirical basis for these recommendations is given.

Another report stating that LSD elicits abreaction and intensifies transference reactions has been published by Rolo et al. (1964). In their procedure, three therapists were present during the LSD experience. According to the authors, one therapist was almost invariably selected as a parental figure or "protector," another as the "enemy." The patient frequently moved spontaneously into highly traumatic childhood experiences. Greater success was reported with patients who had previously been in analysis than with "relatively psychologically unsophisticated" patients. In contrast to Baker (1964), these authors employed a dose of only 100 μg of LSD. They report that a large dose inhibits rather than enhances the response pattern desired. Clearly, if the utility of LSD in an analytic context is accepted, controlled studies are required which hold sophistication, setting, and therapists constant while varying the LSD dosage experimentally. This is one of many examples of the sort of researchable question that arises in the treatment literature, but which does not seem to be undergoing adequate investigation. In the study by Rolo *et al.* (1964) the LSD interview was terminated, after 4 to 5 hours, with phenothiazines or barbiturates. Of the 47 patients treated in this way, 85 per cent claimed improvement and 64 per cent were judged by the staff to have improved. After-care is considered very important, as the authors report that follow-up studies of patients not receiving such care (presumably not the 47 reported here) showed a very high relapse rate.

Chandler and Hartman (1960) reported on a series of 110 patients given LSD as part of a psychoanalytically oriented program. These patients were largely neurotics, or were suffering from personality or sociopathic disorders. They received an average of six LSD sessions, ranging from one session to twenty-six. Dosage was gradually increased, in successive sessions, from 50 to 150 μg. Patients were told, in detail, what might occur under LSD and were given a brief description of the unconscious and its "language of symbolism"; they were also given specific examples of the kind of experience they might have. The drug was given in the room where the patient regularly received psychotherapy and the patient was encouraged to lie on a couch and keep his eyes closed. External stimuli were kept to a minimum. Judgments of outcome were based on symptomatic change, reports from family and friends, evidence of behavioral change in handling real-life problems, productivity, tolerance of anxiety in continuing therapy, and the patient's subjective report. Approximately two-thirds of the patients were reported to have shown improvement. About 45 per cent were considerably improved. In this study, LSD was used in a context of psychoanalysis which continued before and after the LSD sessions for most patients. The authors state that 69 per cent definitely made more rapid progress in conventional therapy as a result of the LSD sessions.

Sandison (1954) emphasizes the abreactive qualities of LSD as the basis for its utility in treatment, but from a Jungian rather than a Freudian point of view. Under the influence of LSD unconscious material, including the archetypal, is said to become available to consciousness but it must be dealt with in a therapeutic setting. Sandison's procedure involved repeated sessions with dosage gradually increased from 25 to 200 μg at approximately weekly intervals (Sandison, Spencer, and Whitelaw, 1954). A modification of the procedure was made with later patients by adding pentobarbital to terminate the LSD effects and reduce anxiety, and by giving chlorpromazine to prevent a recurrence of LSD experiences. Severe anxiety appears to be common in the use of the drug for its abreactive effects, judging from the frequent inclusion in the procedures of measures to calm the patient, or to protect him from his own agitation (Baker, 1964). Sandison and Whitelaw (1957) reported their results with a total of 100 patients. Thirty-six of these were followed up after more than two years had elapsed. Of the latter, 19 were assessed as improved at the latest follow-up. Of the total series followed up after various lengths of time 61 were reported as recovered or improved. The cases included psychoneurotics, psychopaths, and patients suffering personality disorders.

Ling and Buckman (1960) reported the results of LSD-aided psychotherapy with 50 patients suffering from neuroses and character disorders. Dosages for these patients were built up, in successive sessions, to 100 μg in most cases, but as high as 200 μg in some. Metamphetamine was given to alleviate anxiety, and each session was terminated with Mellaril or chlorpromazine. LSD is said to have facilitated the reliving of repressed experiences (even dating to early childhood). Evaluation, six months after the beginning of treatment, showed 38 patients somewhat improved, and 15 of these showed recovery or great improvement. The patients spent one night a week in a psychiatric night hospital where they received LSD and they continued to work during the rest of the week.

Eisner and Cohen (1958) administered LSD to 22 neurotic patients in doses increasing from 25 to 125 μg in weekly sessions. One therapist was always present throughout the LSD session; at times, two were present. The assessments of two therapists and one person in close contact with the patients were employed in rating improvement and were made after a minimum of 6 months. Sixteen patients were considered to have improved.

Martin (1957) administered LSD to 50 patients, largely neurotics, during psychoanalytic therapy. In from two to twenty repeated sessions the dose was increased from 25 to a maximum of 450 μg (or until an "optimal reaction" was obtained). Each session was terminated with chlorpromazine. Forty-six patients showed at least slight improvement, while 19 were cured or markedly improved. After two years, nine cases had relapsed.

Butterworth (1962) treated 52 patients who had failed to progress in psychoanalytically oriented psychotherapy on an outpatient basis. The degree of improvement was related to a "philosophical approach to life" or to curiosity and a need to search for truth. This report is unusual in that some benefit is claimed for all 52 patients. Nine of these were only slightly improved; 13 were "cured."

Ball and Armstrong (1961) reported on the use of LSD with ten patients with various sexual perversions. Their techniques involved a single dose of 200 μg of LSD, administered the day following admission to a psychiatric ward. Preparation for LSD was limited to a single interview preceding the day of treatment, during which the treatment was explained and the patient reassured. The therapists were present during the LSD session, but were relatively inactive. The patients were discharged after one day of observation. During the LSD session, "intense, almost unbearable insight" was often apparent. Two patients are reported to have shown marked subsequent improvement. One of these showed primarily an intense mystical experience with little abreaction during the LSD session; the other, just the reverse. In both cases, but particularly in the latter, considerable negative affect

32

was experienced. The other eight patients claimed improvement, but the authors felt that these claims were not justified by their subsequent behavior. The authors suggest that, as in any type of psychotherapy, above average intelligence and genuine motivation to change are critical factors in a favorable response.

Tenenbaum (1961) and Spencer (1963) have both reported on the use of LSD in group psychotherapy. Tenenbaum's group consisted of ten patients suffering from character disorders. The goal of treatment was symptomatic relief and behavior change rather than radical personality alteration. Only one patient failed to respond favorably. Spencer (1963) employed the transference paradigm in therapy with a group of ten neurotics and patients with character disorders. Doctor and nurse acted as parent surrogates during these sessions, which were held twice a week for 16 months. Three patients improved to the point where they required no further psychiatric help, four others improved noticeably, and three were unimproved.

There are also a number of less detailed reports of LSD treatment. For example, Giberti, Gregoretti, and Boeri (1956) found good to excellent improvement in 17 of 35 neurotics given 30 to 200 μg of LSD. Fontana (1961) reports that, of 88 patients (psychoneurotics and those with character disorders) given "prolonged" treatment with 100 μg of LSD, 22 were cured, 28 much improved, 19 improved, and 19 unchanged. Another series of 78 patients given "short-term" treatment (Fontana, 1961) showed 9 cured, 34 much improved, 25 improved, and 10 unchanged. Vanggaard (1965) treated 22 patients with LSD, of whom 5 showed considerable improvement, 4 improvement to a lesser degree, and 13 no change or deterioration. Arendsen-Hein (1961) treated 21 criminal psychopaths with LSD, of whom 14 showed improvement. With these psychopaths LSD reduced resistance, revealed conflicts, and increased introspection and insight.

The treatment studies summarized above were undertaken either in a psychoanalytic or in an eclectic context. Sherwood, Stolaroff, and Harman (1962) emphasize the unique qualities of the experiences possible under LSD rather than the facilitation of phenomena encountered in ordinary psychotherapy. They delineate three stages of the LSD reaction—an evasive stage, a symbolic stage, and a stage of immediate perception. The latter is the goal of their treatment. During this stage, the patient is said to undergo complete revitalization of the self-concept.

Sherwood, Stolaroff, and Harman (1962) reported the results of LSD treatment with this psychedelic orientation for 25 patients, including seven neurotics and a variety of persons suffering personality disorders. The patients received a single dose of 100 to 200 μg of LSD, supplemented when necessary by from 200 to 400 mg of mescaline. Twelve patients are said to have improved considerably, nine were somewhat improved, and four showed no improvement.

Another study with the "psychedelic" orientation is presented by Savage *et al.* (1965). This study stands out because the investigators used standard psychological tests before and after treatment, in addition to the usual clinical evaluations and patients' claims, in the assessment of outcomes. The clinical evaluations themselves were careful and detailed and for these reasons this study merits fuller examination.

There were 77 patients treated, two-thirds of whom were neurotics or suffered character disorders. One-third were characterized as "normal depressives"—complaining of lack of purpose, lack of meaning in life, or a sense of lack of fulfillment. All patients were selected from volunteers for the program and they paid the medical costs of the treatment. Forty per cent of the applicants were rejected for LSD treatment for a variety of reasons including overt psychosis, severe depression, cardiovascular disease, unsettled life circumstances, and poor motivation. The final 77 patients, therefore, were a special sample, which included a large number of people who were not in any great need of psychiatric treatment.

Those selected were seen for weekly interviews for four to five weeks preceding the LSD session. At these preparatory interviews, autobiographies written by the patients, and patients' expectations of treatment were discussed. Toward the end of each interview, the patient was given inhalations of a CO_2–O_2 mixture to provide experience of transient dissociation without loss of consciousness, and to develop trust and confidence in the therapist. The LSD session took place in the presence of two therapists, who provided "companionship but not interpretation." The dose of LSD was 200–300 μg, supplemented if necessary by 200–300 mg of mescaline sulphate. Pupillary dilation was used as the index of an adequate dose. Patients were interviewed the next day, and 1, 4, 8, 12, and 24 weeks later. The final evaluation of the 77 patients was made after six months.

A global rating by the entire staff based on all available data (psychological tests, therapist's ratings, interview by independent judges) was made for 76 out of the 77 patients, and the lowest rating prevailed. By this criterion, 12 showed marked improvement, 22 moderate improvement, 28 minimal improvement, and 14 no improvement or deterioration. Sixty patients completed the testing program. On a value-belief Q- sort, there were significant increases after LSD treatment in endorsement of test items reflecting open-mindedness, a sense of purpose, and unity with nature and humanity. Stable, positive changes occurred in MMPI profiles. On the Interpersonal Check-list, there were significant increases in self-assertiveness and confidence, but no significant over-all changes on the *Love* scale. Several positive changes were indicated in the Behavior Change Interview, consisting of 433 items and administered 6 months following the LSD experience.

The authors correctly comment that the generality of the findings is limited by the selection process. This is true of the other studies summarized as well, where in most cases the selection process is not specified in the detail provided here.

An unusual study by Ditman, Hayman, and Whittlesey (1962) found LSD effects in a non-treatment setting. This study was conducted in a "permissive and enthusiastic but non-treatment setting." The subjects were volunteers who had come with the expectation of an interesting and perhaps worthwhile experience. They were given LSD as part of a study comparing the LSD and delirium tremens experiences. The subjects included colleagues and acquaintances of the investigators, alcoholics, and neurotics. The dose was 100 μg. This group was given a 12-page questionnaire from six months to two years following the LSD experience. Forty-nine (66 per cent) of the 74 subjects responding to the questionnaire claimed some improvement as a result of LSD; 49 per cent claimed moderate to substantial improvement in their feelings. Thus, in this study, with no deliberate therapeutic aims, and with a sample, half of which consisted of normals who volunteered out of curiosity alone, an incidence of claimed improvement comparable with that found in the psychiatric studies was obtained. As the authors suggest, "perhaps LSD is unique in that it promotes many claims, not only from subjects and patients, but from investigators themselves."

It might be added that in most of the studies summarized to this point, the therapists have had a personal LSD experience. In fact, this is often said to be highly desirable if not essential for effective therapeutic use of the drug (e.g., Eisner and Cohen, 1958). However, there may be real danger that assessments of outcome of the drug may be influenced by the therapist's commitment to a belief in its unique effects, reinforced by his own experience. Ditman, Hayman, and Whittlesey (1962) reported that mystics, compared to members of the three large religious groups and to agnostics, claimed the most for the LSD experience. McGlothlin, Cohen, and McGlothlin (1964) found that positive attitudes toward LSD are associated with more introverted and intuitive scores on a test constructed to measure Jungian personality types, and with higher hypnotic susceptibility.

These and other similar findings suggest the possibility that enthusiasm for LSD (before its effects are experienced, but given the widespread publicity the drug has received) may often reflect a need for an unusual experience and a strong inclination to interpret it in mystical and far-reaching terms, both in subjects and patients who seek out the opportunity to take the drug and in the therapists themselves. There are many social psychological studies showing the effects of behavioral commitment on attitudes following the commitment (Festinger, 1957; Brehm and Cohen, 1962). Attitudes change in directions justifying the commitment in situations where the individual perceives that he has a choice. Particularly in a study like that of Savage et al. (1965) summarized above, where the patients are volunteers, where they know that they must pass a fairly rigorous screening process (40 per cent of the volunteers were not accepted for treatment), and where they must agree to bear the costs of treatment, some of the positive claims, and even some of the changes on standard tests that depend on self-report, may be accounted for in these terms. A further possibility is that commitment to or an expectation of certain drug effects makes these effects possible. Such considerations also apply, of course, to any other form of treatment.

A report by Whitaker (1964a, 1964b) is apparently unique in that the therapist deliberately refrained from taking LSD before using it in therapy. Whitaker's study is of special interest, also, in that it compares the outcome of the LSD treatment group with the outcome of a comparable group who did not receive LSD. The LSD group was composed of 100 patients—neurotics and persons with sexual and personality disorders. A control group was collected from patients with a comparable range of diagnoses and similar duration of illness who had been treated before the introduction of LSD. In Whitaker's study (1964a, 1964b) LSD treatment was combined with ordinary psychotherapy. Prior to receiving LSD, the patients were instructed in the effects of the drug and advised not to resist them. The dose was between 100 and 250 μg and the experience was terminated by the administration of chlorpromazine. During the session the therapist was active in encouraging abreactive experiences and their integration. Psychotherapy was continued between LSD sessions, which ranged from 1 to 10 in number. The criteria for improvement were relief of symptoms and insight. Outcome was assessed by the investigator.

Forty-seven LSD patients either recovered or were much improved. These patients showed complete, or almost complete relief from symptoms in addition to insight. Eighteen were somewhat improved, and 35 were unimproved. The last group includes those who evaded treatment after one session. The outcomes in the control group of 100 patients were 12 recovered or much improved, 30 somewhat improved, and 58 unimproved. A detailed analysis of outcomes is provided in relation to diagnosis, duration of illness, type of LSD reaction, and "level of regression" (the earliest age from which experiences were recalled under LSD). The most striking of the findings reported here was the high incidence of complete failure (20 of 21 cases) in patients who "intellectualized" the experience. Only one patient in this series experienced ecstasy or pleasant affect under LSD.

Only one study was encountered in the literature (Robinson, Davies, Sack, and Morrissey, 1963) in which patients were randomly assigned to LSD or comparison groups. The patients in this study were selected from a population of in-patients at an institution for the short-term treatment of neurotics. The general treatment facilities at this institution included a variety of social activities, group discussions about the running of the center, and group occupational therapy and physical training. All patients who were at least average in intelligence and between 18 and 35 years of age were considered for the treatment experiment. On the basis of diagnostic interviews patients were excluded on a variety of grounds, including organic disorders, a psychotic history, obsessional neuroses, and personality disorders. Those patients who were eligible by the initial criteria and who were not excluded on other grounds were randomly assigned to one of three groups.

Thirty-three were assigned to "standard therapy," of whom 26 completed treatment. This consisted of individual psychotherapy, including reassurance, support, suggestion, and encouragement to ventilate feelings and gain insight into symptoms and their relation to the patient's current situation. No pharmacological agent was employed to encourage abreaction. Thirty-five patients were assigned to LSD therapy, and 33 completed the treatment. These patients were given an initial dose of 50 μg of LSD increased weekly by 25 μg, and each session was terminated by chlorpromazine after six hours. During the LSD session, the patient was in bed in a single room, and was encouraged to let his mind wander and to talk about his experiences. Thirty-three patients were assigned to Cyclonal and Methedrine therapy, and 28 completed the treatment. The purpose of this treatment was to provide a comparison with LSD of a drug combination which also, in the author's experience, facilitated abreaction. The drug combination was given at weekly intervals, the therapist remaining with the patient for at least one hour after administration.

Patients failed to complete the assigned treatments for a variety of reasons, reportedly extraneous to the research. The full course of treatment in each case was eight weeks. Patients were assessed clinically before treatment. They were assessed again immediately following treatment, and at three and six months after discharge. At the second assessment, immediately after treatment, ratings were made by an independent psychiatrist without knowledge of the treatment each patient had received. Using a criterion of freedom from symptoms, 62 per cent of the standard group, 60 per cent of the LSD group, and 50 per cent of the Methedrine group had benefited from treatment. Eighty-nine per cent of the standard, 79 per cent of the LSD and 79 per cent of the Methedrine group showed at least some improvement. Differences among the three groups are not sufficient with either criterion.

The six-month and three-month assessments were made by the patients' own doctors—either the referring psychiatrist or general practitioner or both. At six months, 11 of 21 patients reporting in the standard group were symptom-free and well-adjusted, but 16 of 23 in the LSD group, and 12 of 21 in the Methedrine group were symptom-free. The differences between the groups were not statistically significant. Thus, there was no clear evidence for a superiority of LSD over the two other methods of treatment. Immediately following treatment, the evidence favored standard psychotherapy over LSD. Six months after treatment, but with a substantially reduced sample for which data were available, LSD appeared to be superior. In both cases, however, the null hypothesis of no difference between treatments could not be rejected with any confidence.

Table I summarizes the outcomes of treatment with LSD for the 20 studies reviewed, including the report by Robinson *et al.* Outcomes reported for other types of treatment are presented in Table II. There are, of course, many ways in which these reports are not strictly comparable: they vary in the length and thoroughness of follow-up; in the diagnostic composition of the patients treated; in the form of treatment, including the details of the LSD session or sessions, the amount and kind of preparation, the amount of psychotherapy without LSD; in the criteria for improvement; and in many other ways. All one can say about the variation in outcome is that it is not related in any obvious way to the methodological variation, and that a very wide variety of methods has been tried.

If all reports are combined, 785 of 1089 (71 per cent) patients

TABLE I

SUMMARY: OUTCOME OF TREATMENT WITH LSD

Source	Total number of patients	Improved or benefited by treatment in any degree		Markedly improved or recovered	
		Number	(% total)	Number	(% total)
Baker (1964)	150	100	(67)	8[a]	(5)%
Chandler & Hartman (1960)	110	73	(66)	50	(45)
Whitaker (1964)					
LSD group	100	65	(65)	47	(47)
Sandison & Whitlaw (1957)	100	61	(61)	—[a]	—[a]
Fontana (1961)					
"long-term"	88	69	(78)	50	(57)
"short-term"	78	68	(87)	43	(55)
Savage et al. (1965)	76	62	(82)	34	(45)
Butterworth (1962)	52	52	(100)	43	(83)
Martin (1957)	50	46	(92)	19	(38)
Ling & Buckman (1960)	50	38	(76)	15	(30)
Rolo et al. (1964)	47	30	(64)	—[a]	—[a]
Giberti et al. (1956)	35	17	(48)	—[a]	—[a]
Robinson et al. (1963)					
LSD group	33	26[b]	(79)	20[b]	(60)
Sherwood et al. (1962)	25	21	(84)	12	(48)
Vanggaard (1965)	22	9	(41)	5	(23)
Eisner & Cohen (1958)	22	16	(73)	—[a]	—[a]
Arendsen-Hein (1961)	21	14	(67)	—[a]	—[a]
Ball & Armstrong (1961)	10	2	(20)	2	(20)
Tenenbaum (1961)	10	9	(90)	—[a]	—[a]
Spencer (1963)	10	7	(70)	3	(30)
ALL REPORTS COMBINED	1089	785	(71%)	351	(45%[c])
Ditman et al. (1962): LSD without therapeutic intent	74	49	(66%)	36	(49%)

[a]Information not reported.
[b]Immediately following treatment.
[c]Percentage of 785 patients in those reports where information available.

TABLE II

OUTCOME OF SELECTED COMPARISON TREATMENTS NOT INVOLVING LSD

Source	Total number of patients	Improved or benefited in any degree		Markedly improved or recovered	
		Number	(% total)	Number	(% total)
Whitaker (1964)					
control group	100	42	(42)	12	(12)
Robinson et al. (1963)					
standard therapy	26	23	(89)	16	(62)
cyclonal–Methedrine	28	22	(79)	14	(50)
Eysenck (1961)					
Total of 5 reports of outcome of psycho-analytic treatment	760	496	(65)	335	(44)

improved after LSD at least to some degree. In those studies where it is possible to make the distinction, 45 per cent of the patients treated improved markedly or were totally free of symptoms. Eleven of the 20 studies report between 60 and 80 per cent of the patients treated at least somewhat improved. Robinson *et al.* (1963) report 79 per cent improved immediately after treatment, and 70 per cent of those contacted after six months were still improved. Thus the results of their LSD therapy are fairly typical of those reported by other authors who included no control group; and Robinson *et al.* (1963) found no significant difference between the LSD group and their two control groups.

It is interesting, also, to compare the proportion of patients improved after LSD treatment in all studies with the improvement claimed by the subjects in the research of Ditman, Hayman, and Whittlesey (1962). In this study there was no therapeutic intention, and, in fact, a substantial number of subjects had no serious psychiatric problem, so far as was known. The percentage of these subjects claiming improvement to some degree (66 per cent) is within the modal range reported in the studies where the intent was clearly therapeutic.

Eysenck (1961) reviewed the results of studies (not involving LSD) reporting improvement in neurotics, and in patients suffering other non-psychotic, functional psychiatric disorders. In five studies (without control groups) of the outcome of psychoanalytic treatment, 65 per cent of the patients were improved to some degree on follow-up. This is not clearly inferior to the incidence of improvement reported in the LSD studies.

These comparisons cast some doubt on the special efficacy of LSD in producing improvement in neurotic patients. Only Whitaker (1964a, 1964b) found it to be superior by direct comparison to other, unspecified forms of treatment, but his control group was constructed from files after collection of the LSD cases, rather than by random assignment from the same population.

We can conclude, then, that the effectiveness of LSD in psychotherapy with non-psychotic psychiatric patients has not been clearly demonstrated. This conclusion follows, basically, from the failure of many investigators using LSD in treatment to meet the minimal requirements for an objective assessment of the value of LSD in therapy, combined with the negative results where these requirements have been met. Even accepting at face value the claims of LSD therapists, those comparisons that can be made with other types of psychotherapy show no clear superiority for LSD. The presence or absence of various details in therapeutic procedure with LSD which are claimed by one writer or another to be important to its effectiveness shows no clear relationship to the percentage of favorable outcomes.

3. LSD in the Treatment of Alcoholism

EFFECTS OF LSD ON DRINKING BEHAVIOR

A NUMBER OF OBSERVERS HAVE COMMENTED on the low scientific standards which prevail in the clinical trials of new drugs. (Foulds, 1958; Glick and Margolis, 1962). The lack of control groups, follow-up procedures, and objective measurements of change has characterized psychiatric research on both pharmacological and psychological treatment methods (Eysenck, 1960; Meehl, 1955). This general lack of sophistication is especially characteristic of the attempts to examine the effectiveness of LSD-25 (d-lysergic acid diethylamide) as an adjunct to the treatment of alcoholism. Several groups of investigators have reported clinical trials in which LSD was alleged to be effective in treating alcoholism, but the reports of many such trials are little more than the chronicling of clinical procedure. The rate of improvement in alcoholism due to LSD therapy varies greatly from one study to another, about 60 per cent being close to the average.

The reported range of improvement and abstinence rates is very wide for alcoholics treated with LSD. Smith (1958) reported that 12 out of 24 alcoholics were "improved" or "much improved" in terms of their drinking histories. Later Chwelos et al. (1959) reported 15 out of 16 and MacLean et al. (1961) 46 out of 61 alcoholics "improved" or "much improved" after LSD. In addition, Chandler and Hartman (1960) have reported that a series of LSD sessions created "considerable improvement in 17 alcoholic and/or narcotic addicts," and Eisner and Cohen (1958) found that 2 out of 3 alcoholics given LSD were "improved" although no criteria for these judgments were given. Ditman, Hayman, and Whittlesey (1962) found that LSD given in a non-treatment setting resulted in 67 per cent of their alcoholics stopping or decreasing their drinking. O'Reilly and Reich (1962) found 17 out of 33 alcoholics abstinent or improved. The report by Jensen and Ramsay (1963) states that 63 per cent of alcoholics given LSD in a group setting were abstinent for 6 to 18 months compared with only 27 per cent in a group given individual psychiatric treatment. Fragmentary reports[2] of the effectiveness of LSD with alcoholics have also been made by Whittlesey (Abramson, 1960), Peck (Abramson, 1960), and Savage (1962). These three reports are too brief to allow detailed consideration and will not be referred to in this analysis since they are essentially anecdotal in nature and do not give details about dosage, setting, follow-up procedures, and methods of assessing change.

The important design features of the nine full reports on LSD and alcoholism are summarized in Table III. It has been concluded from these reports that LSD is "effective in the treatment of alcoholism" (e.g., MacLean *et al.*, 1961) and it now comprises a major part of the therapy in several Canadian and American treatment centers for alcoholics. The aim here is to examine closely the studies purporting to show that LSD is a useful adjunct to therapy for alcoholics. A further hope is that the minimal requirements for any drug research in alcoholism will be clarified during the course of the analysis.

The basic requirements for clinical research into the efficacy of any new treatment have been frequently outlined (Eysenck, 1960; Meehl, 1955). They include at least the following procedures. To determine whether a new drug is effective it is necessary to use a control group receiving a placebo or some relatively inert drug. If one does not wish to compare the effects of the new drug with the placebo effects, at least a no-drug control group must be used which gets another form of treatment against which the drug is to be evaluated. There should be a random assignment of patients to the various treatment groups, including the control or placebo groups. All control groups should get identical treatment except for the drug variables to be studied. If placebos are used, the study should be double-blind, i.e., neither the treatment

---

[2]For example, Benedetti (1951) studied the effects of two doses of LSD on one alcoholic. The text of this paper has not been seen and the abstract does not clearly indicate the control methods used.

personnel nor the patient may know which drug the latter receives. Finally, some objective measures or uncontaminated ratings[3] of subjective treatment outcome are required. These measurements should be made both before and after treatment so that pre- and post-treatment comparisons can be made. The post-treatment measures should be part of a follow-up procedure which is undertaken at relatively fixed intervals after treatment.

Table III, summarizing much of the information on methodology employed in studies of LSD and alcoholism, shows that the nine studies do not adhere closely to the basic methodological requirements cited above. For example, only one study has used a control group which received either a placebo or some other form of treatment. This deficiency opens the door to many interpretations of the positive findings. It makes it impossible to state whether the changes in drinking behavior were due to LSD or to such variables as the greater staff interest in the patients during the study (by way of special interviews, questionnaires, follow-up, and the like), or other types of treatment intervention such as Alcoholics Anonymous, private medical care, or social agencies. The lack of control groups also raises the possibility that the positive findings could be attributable to spontaneous recovery. The proportion of alcoholics likely to recover spontaneously is unknown at present but isolated cases do occur.

The only study employing a "control" is the one by Jensen and Ramsay (1963), but what was being controlled is difficult to determine. Ideally, the control treatment should duplicate as many of the features of the LSD treatment as possible—without administration of LSD. In this study the control group received individual out-patient treatment by psychiatrists, whereas the LSD group got a two-month period of group psychotherapy as in-patients, together with a single LSD session. The method of assignment to treatment groups is not stated, and it is not clear that patients in the two groups were similar in any important respects. Clearly, the Jensen and Ramsay study does not provide the type of control needed.

[3]That is, uncontaminated by the raters' knowledge of what treatment the patient received.

TABLE III

THE METHODOLOGICAL FEATURES OF STUDIES PURPORTING TO SHOW LSD TO BE A USEFUL ADJUNCT TO THE TREATMENT OF ALCOHOLISM

Authors	Number and type of alcoholics	Dose	Placebo control	Other control	Pre-treatment measures	Post-treatment measures	Length of follow-up
1. Smith (1958)	24 male alcoholics mainly diagnosed as psychopaths or suffering character disorders	200–400 μg (1 or 2 sessions)	None	None	Not stated	Some material on drinking but exact nature not stated	2 mo. to 3 yr.
2. Eisner & Cohen (1958)	3 male alcoholics with chronic anxiety states	25–150 mg (4–6 sessions)	None	None	Not stated	Reports on drinking and adjustment obtained from patient and someone in close contact with him	6 to 17 mo.
3. Chwelos et al. (1959)	16 alcoholics mainly diagnosed as psychopaths or suffering character disorders	200–400 μg (number of sessions unstated)	None	None	Not stated	Reports on drinking from A.A. contacts with the the patient, and his family	2 to 9 mo.
4. Chandler and Hartman (1960)	17 alcohol and/or narcotic addicts (not differentiated)	Not stated (1–26 sessions)	None	None	Not stated	Reports from family and friends, improvement in symptom picture, manner and bearing during therapy; patients subjective report of his degree of improvement	No follow-up
5. MacLean et al. (1961)	50 male and 11 female alcoholics mainly diagnosed as sociopathic and with personality trait disturbances	400–1500 μg (1 session)	None	None	Autobiography; psychiatric history and notes; clinical examination	Record of post-treatment period of counselling; patients description of LSD experience; Blewett's Psychedelic	3 to 18 mo.

				including certain unstated blood chemistry tests	A Scale; Psychiatrist's immediate post-treatment impressions; notes from psychiatric interviews—1 week and 3 mo. after; Blewett's Psychedelic B Scale; undescribed follow-up data collected by counselors; an undisclosed questionnaire completed 6 mo. after therapy; a psychiatric interview and appraisal at the end of 1 year	
6. Ditman, Hayman, & Whittlesey (1962)	27 alcoholics	100 μg (1 or more sessions)	None	None	Not stated	Questionnaire completed by patients	1½ to 3 yr.
7. Jensen & Ramsay (1963)	70 alcoholics	200 μg (1 session)	None	55 alcoholics admitted to individual treatment by psychiatrists	Not stated	Not clearly stated but some reports on drinking	6 to 18 mo. 62 LSD follow-ups but only 29 of the controls
8. O'Reilly and Funk (1964)	68 alcoholics (non-psychotic)	200 μg (1 session)	None	None	Not stated	Questionnaires completed by patient, friends, or relatives on drinking	2 to 34 mo.
9. O'Reilly and Reich (1962)	33 alcoholics	200 μg (1 or 2 sessions)	None	None	Not stated	Questionnaire given to patients. Reports from relatives and treatment agencies	7 to 88 weeks

Unfortunately, the absence of control groups in research on new psychiatric treatments seems to be the rule rather than the exception. To illustrate, Foulds (1958) found that 72 per cent of the research studies of new treatments reported in psychiatric journals (1951–1956) lacked controls. Moreover, he found that 83 per cent of the uncontrolled studies, but only 25 per cent of the controlled studies, reported that the treatments were successful. In addition, Glick and Margolis (1962), after reviewing the literature on chlorpromazine, found significantly lower clinical improvement rates in double-blind controlled studies than in non-blind uncontrolled ones. There is some basis, then, for expecting non-blind uncontrolled studies, such as those discussed here, to yield a considerably higher number of positive results. The larger proportion of positive results in uncontrolled studies exists despite the lack of the very elements of design which would allow any firm conclusion.

The lack of double-blind or even single-blind procedures also raises the possibility that the reported effects of LSD are attributable in part to the patients' expectations about the drug rather than to its pharmacological action. All of the patients in the LSD studies reported were aware that this drug was being administered, as were the therapists. As in other drug research, placebo reactors have been found in studies of the physiological and psychological effects of LSD (Abramson, Jarvik, Levine, Kaufman, and Hirsch, 1955; Abramson, Jarvik, Kaufman, Kornetsky, Levine, and Wagner, 1955) and many of their symptoms correspond to the real effects of LSD. Whether the mere belief that an LSD experience was obtained is sufficient to account for or add to the positive results cannot be answered. It would be reassuring to have these doubts dispelled by results showing that placebo effects were unimportant in LSD therapy. The possibility that placebo effects might be important is also supported by the impression that alcoholics with character disorders or psychopathy are most improved by treatment with LSD (Smith, 1958; Chwelos *et al.*, 1959). It has been reported that placebo reactors score high on psychological tests of neuroticism and extroversion (Knowles and Lucas, 1960; Joyce, 1961) and these characteristics are found in persons with psychopathic disturbances and character disorders (Eysenck, 1957). The similarities between the personality characteristics of placebo reactors and those who respond most favorably to LSD at least suggests that placebo responses might partially account for the response to this drug. All of the above considerations tend to raise doubt concerning the effectiveness of LSD as an adjunct to therapy for alcoholism.

Certain criticisms have been made of double-blind trials but none of them seem convincing. For example, it has been argued by Haas, Fink, and Hartfelder (1959) that ethical doubts are raised when the physician does not know what drug is being administered to his patient. However, ethical questions are also raised when physicians administer drugs whose effects have not been scientifically validated, or when they persist in applying treatments with unknown or uncertain outcomes. Double-blind trials, used with proper controls, are designed to reduce ignorance about new treatments and are justified on that basis alone. Haas, Fink, and Hartfelder also suggested that complicated double-blind trials create the possibility of errors in the analysis of the results, and that such trials are difficult to plan. There seems to be no argument against this objection except to state that the possibility of error and the difficulties of design do not outweigh the values of such studies. A more telling criticism is that "blindness" in placebo-controlled studies may be difficult to achieve when testing drugs with strong sensory effects, such as LSD. However, double-blind trials of LSD could surely be done with a placebo having some immediate but mild sensory effects. The sensory and perceptual effects of LSD vary markedly from person to person, so that patients given a placebo might have a drug experience not unlike that reported by some persons who actually receive LSD. This would be the case particularly where patients did not know that LSD was being used. It would be possible to keep the trials "blind" by reminding all patients in the study that the effects of the drugs being given are highly variable, even to the point of creating almost no reaction. Whether experienced LSD therapists could be deceived about which patients received the drug is difficult to say; probably many could not.

Non-blind uncontrolled trials have also been defended as indicating which drugs might repay more careful investigation and controlled study. In the great race to produce more drugs and more treatments for mental disorders, sufficient time to evaluate them is often not taken.[4] The testing of a drug in uncontrolled trials does not necessarily establish it as a promising therapeutic measure. In fact, it may mean, as with LSD, that clinical use is made of the drug before its real effectiveness is properly assessed.

The only methodological requirement met in many LSD studies is the follow-up procedure, but even this is vulnerable to criticism. The study by Chandler and Hartman (1960) gives no indication of any post-treatment follow-up. Eisner and Cohen (1958) mention that follow-up was conducted 6 to 17 months after therapy, but there is no inkling of what material was gathered, or how it was used in assessing recovery. The studies by Smith (1958), Chwelos et al. (1959), Jensen and Ramsay (1963), O'Reilly and Funk (1964), and O'Reilly and Reich (1962) refer to follow-up information collected at varying intervals after treatment, but the type of information collected is not described. Apparently, descriptions of drinking experiences after treatment were obtained in order to categorize patients as "much improved," "improved," or "unchanged." Unfortunately, neither the exact information sought nor the sources from which it was sought were reported. It is not known, for example, whether statements about post-treatment drinking were obtained from both patients and relatives, or what weight was given to the various reports if they conflicted. A further problem with these studies is the lack of objective or uncontaminated subjective information for the pre-treatment period. If a detailed drinking history was sought only during follow-up, then the patient's expectations of change, especially in a non-blind study, might confuse fact and fiction in the information he gives.

The study by MacLean et al. (1961) does describe certain types of pre-treatment information, obtained chiefly by way of an auto-biography, a psychiatric history, and certain chemical tests.

[4]In this connection the review of the effectiveness of the somatotherapies by Staudt and Zubin (1957) is especially relevant.

However, these pre-treatment measures appear to be different from those in the post-treatment follow-ups. Apparently, psychiatric interviews were held and psychiatric assessments made one week, three months, and one year after treatment; an undisclosed "questionnaire" was administered; and certain follow-up data concerning interpersonal relationships, work habits, and self-appraisals were obtained. But nowhere is there any clear indication that the data solicited, pre- and post-treatment, were identical or even similar. Consequently, follow-up constituted a post-therapy study with few pre-therapy measures which could be correlated, except for the psychiatric assessments.

A further problem in all of these studies relates to the very wide range of intervals at which follow-up was done: 2 months to 3 years in Smith's study (1958), 3 to 18 months in the MacLean *et al.* study (1961), 6 to 17 months in the Eisner and Cohen study (1958), 2 to 34 months in the O'Reilly and Funk study (1964), 6 to 18 months in the Jensen and Ramsay study (1963), 2 to 9 months in that by Chwelos *et al.* (1959), and 7 to 88 weeks in the O'Reilly and Reich (1962) study. In all of these studies, but particularly in the first two, the range of post-treatment opportunities for the alcoholics to resume drinking is extremely wide. It does not seem reasonable to lump patients with two months of follow-up with those having three years of follow-up. This problem becomes further complicated when it is realized that the numbers of alcoholics rated "much improved" and "improved" in terms of social adjustment, personality adjustment, and drinking history vary markedly with the length of follow-up (Wallerstein, 1957). Wallerstein's comparison (1957) of disulfiram, hypnotherapy, conditioned reflex, and milieu therapy seems to show that the percentage of improved patients varies over the range of follow-up intervals from 6 to 24 months. The percentage of "improved" cases increases with increasing duration of follow-up for all treatments but milieu therapy, and for the latter this percentage decreases. What the relationship is for LSD therapy is impossible to say from the available data, except that the very large variation could produce several sets of relationships. Unambiguous interpretation of treatment outcome studies demands comparable estimates of pre- and post-treatment behavior and a relatively constant follow-up period.

The arguments presented above are sufficient to raise serious questions concerning the scientific warrant for any belief that LSD is a useful adjunct to the treatment of alcoholism. The purpose here is not to argue that it has no effect, but solely to show that the Scottish verdict of "not proven" is the only one justified by the evidence. Further studies involving the requirements discussed above *might* show LSD to be the best available treatment for alcoholism. In fairness to the authors of the LSD reports, it should be noted that most of them made pleas for more clinical trials, although controlled trials were specifically called for only by Smith (1959). Uncontrolled trials alone would never help to decide the effectiveness of any treatment. For these reasons, a double-blind controlled study of the therapeutic usefulness of LSD is required; moreover, results from studies of this general type represent the only ground for hope in the future effective treatment of alcoholism.

Smith (1964) has defended the LSD trials made so far and has commented on some of the methodological criticisms of LSD research. He appears to accept most of the methodological criticisms, but claims that (1) LSD research is poorly financed and hence should be kindly dealt with, (2) this research is not much worse than other treatment research, and (3) research with LSD is still in a very early stage, where the goals are different and the standards applied above are too rigorous and perhaps unnecessary. The first two points, if true, are unfortunate, but would appear to be irrelevant. The claim that LSD research is still in an exploratory phase needs more careful examination.

Concern with the need for an exploratory phase in drug research is readily appreciated. This is a phase in which criticism should be minimized and exploration of all relevant hypotheses maximized. Few would argue against the need for such phases. During the exploratory phase the basic toxic effects and side effects of a drug should be completely investigated, together with the possibilities for its addition to the treatment armamentarium. However, there is a constant danger that the exploratory period will be too short, that too few human subjects will be studied sufficiently well to make valid conclusions possible, and that strong pressure for new treatments will mean that the drug will be used therapeutically before its effects are adequately understood. Once a drug becomes established as a therapeutic agent its real dangers may never be realized until it provokes some catastrophic event such as the well-known thalidomide tragedy. A minimum expectation is that during the exploratory period efforts be made to find out whether the new drug is better than existing treatments and under what conditions its advantages are best realized.

Research with LSD in the treatment of alcoholism has fallen prey to most of the "exploratory phase" dangers listed above. So far, no one has taken the trouble to explore the possibility that its addition to current treatment programs does not produce any changes in drinking other than those which the programs alone produce. In many quarters, especially Saskatchewan and British Columbia, the "exploratory" period with LSD has been over for some time, without providing any satisfactory answers to questions about its efficacy. Also, the "exploratory" period was very brief and far more concerned with therapy than with exploration.

In Saskatchewan, for years the locus of the greatest LSD interest, the exploratory period for its use in alcoholism was extremely short. An interim report by the Bureau on Alcoholism in 1962 gave the official position of the Saskatchewan Department of Health and Welfare: "such excellent results have been noted . . . that LSD treatment which was originally regarded by the Bureau as experimental, *became a standard form of treatment to be used where indicated*" (Bureau on Alcoholism, 1962, italics supplied). When this report appeared just two studies of LSD in the treatment of alcoholics treated in Saskatchewan had been published and only 40 alcoholics were included in them. The interim report is based on the results of LSD therapy with 145 alcoholics,[5] but details of the treatments, follow-up procedures, and methods of evaluation are too vaguely stated to constitute scientific reporting. The report of the Bureau on Alcoholism clearly removed LSD

[5]Perhaps some of these 145 were subsequently reported on by Jensen and Ramsay (1963) and by O'Reilly and Funk (1964).

from the category of "exploratory drug" and established it as an indicated form of treatment for alcoholism—at least in Saskatchewan.

A further difficulty about the exploratory period of LSD research concerns the low ratio of real exploration to actual therapy. The report of the Bureau on Alcoholism gives the impression that LSD was removed from the "experimental" category only at the end of 1962. However, in February 1963 Hoffer reported that more than 500 alcoholics had already been treated in Saskatchewan (quoted in Bureau on Alcoholism, 1963, p. 6). Since only 145 had been involved in any sort of research program, and since data for only 40 were reported in scientific journals, it would appear that LSD was being used as a therapy for some time before the Bureau's report and that only a minority of those alcoholics given LSD were actually participating in any exploratory studies. All of these considerations lead to the conclusion that LSD therapy with alcoholics, at least in Saskatchewan, had by no means a long and painstaking exploratory period. Since it seems clear that LSD was being used as an adjunct to therapy before its effectiveness was established, the nine studies examined above could be subject to criticism.

Minimum standards for studies of LSD have already been presented. These are not original ideas; they represent the application of well-known principles of research design to the evaluation of the effectiveness of LSD treatment of alcoholics. One cannot claim that a study which conformed to these standards would be definitive with respect to *all* questions that might be asked about the treatment being studied, but such a study would be germane to many of the procedural questions as yet unanswered.

As Smith (1964) remarks, we do not yet know what questions to ask about LSD and alcoholism treatment. "LSD treatment" includes more than the administration of the drug and its direct physiological effects, whatever those may be. LSD treatment varies from one institution to another, from one practitioner to another, and from one patient to another. It is nevertheless incumbent on those using the drug (or any other treatment) at any stage of exploration of its effects to conduct their explorations in a way approximating as closely as possible the ideal. Until very recently this had not been done in studies of LSD with alcoholics. To explore the use of a drug treatment not known to be effective, with a disorder like alcoholism where the rate of "improvement" among "untreated" patients is known to be well above zero, one should randomly assign some proportion of candidates for the treatment to a control group which receives only the usual treatment. It is not much more difficult to plan and apply some kind of objective data collection before and after treatment to patients in the experimental and control groups. If 500 alcoholics have been treated with LSD in Saskatchewan, we *should* be in a position to judge confidently whether patients receiving LSD treatment as applied in Saskatchewan are more likely to change in relevant respects than similar patients in Saskatchewan not exposed to such treatment. We are not in this position, and the reason is, apparently, that control groups and objective criteria of change are regarded as appropriate only to a late stage of treatment research.

EFFECTS OF LSD ON PERSONALITY

The general therapeutic effects of LSD have been described in detail in a previous section. The main effects on personality are usually taken to be an uncovering of the unconscious, an integration of ego functions, and a reordering of emotional life. It has also been found that LSD aids during psychoanalysis by removing emotional blocks in the analysis, increasing tolerance to anxiety, and intensifying transference relationships (Abramson, 1960). Of primary interest, here, are the effects of LSD on personality in alcoholics. Many of the studies of LSD therapy in alcoholism have reported major personality changes, especially where a high rate of improvement in drinking was found. These studies have been reviewed in the previous section which was concerned solely with drinking behavior. The methodological difficulties (lack of control groups, of objective pre- and post-measures of change, and of routine follow-ups) that make it difficult to accept the validity of the claims about drinking behavior make it equally difficult to judge the strength of the conclusions about personality change.

55

However, the early studies of LSD therapy and alcoholism have generated a number of interesting and important hypotheses about personality changes. These hypotheses deserve far more careful study than they have received so far, as at present they constitute clinical evaluations of change.

Reports of personality changes in alcoholics are typically based on studies examining only the short-term effects of LSD. For example, MacLean *et al.* (1961) have described the psychedelic experience among alcoholics as marked by "its increased insight, its expanded awareness and its altered frames of reference, that is the therapeutic vehicle." These same authors have also reported that LSD creates a new self-concept which alcoholics find more acceptable, reduces the need for inappropriate defense mechanisms, and reduces anxiety. Chwelos *et al.* (1959) also claimed that LSD therapy removes anxiety and promotes more acceptable self-concepts. In addition they claim that it helps to remove pride, prejudice, guilt, and repression, that it helps the patient to experience a wider range of emotions, to recognize his conflicts more readily, and to develop more sensitivity to the feelings of others. Smith (1959) believes that LSD creates a type of religious conversion involving "a remarkable sense of tranquility and of being at one with the universe." He also supported the proposition that alcoholics treated with LSD show more acceptance of the unpleasant aspects of themselves, can handle conflicts in more constructive ways, and can more readily empathize with others. Savage (1962) found that a large proportion of his alcoholic patients given LSD made claims of "subjective improvement," and of improvement in external factors (e.g., income, abode, occupation) as well as claims of reduced anxiety. Surprisingly, many investigators (e.g., Eisner and Cohen, 1958; Chandler and Hartman, 1960; O'Reilly and Reich, 1962; O'Reilly and Funk, 1964; Jensen and Ramsay, 1963) have not commented on the psychological changes occurring with LSD therapy in alcoholics.

The guesses we have about the psychological effects of LSD on alcoholics come from studies cited in the previous section on drinking behavior, together with a few additional ones. The limitations of these studies have been noted and only a few additional comments are needed here. All claims for psychological effects of LSD in alcoholism rest on clinical studies made without controlled conditions. None of these studies employed untreated or placebo controls whose measured or rated personality changes could be compared with the changes in those given LSD. Also, pre- and post-treatment measurements for evaluating personality changes were not employed, and hence suggestions about personality changes are based solely on unsupported clinical observations. It is possible, as well, that such changes as were reliably observed could have occurred even if LSD had not been administered, since in all cases reported so far LSD was given as an adjunct to more standard therapies, thus making it difficult to know which changes to attribute to LSD and which to the standard therapies.

There can be no argument that the LSD experience is a striking one for many persons, and that it is probably capable of creating or starting personality changes. However, it seems that the strategy of scientific proof has been neglected in establishing what these changes are. The entire area of psychological effects of LSD would benefit greatly from the use of standardized personality tests before and after the LSD experience. So far, these have been used only in studies of the acute effects of LSD rather than in studies of its long-term influence. It is not possible to assume that the acute effects on personality merely become consolidated over time.

EFFECTS OF LSD ON FAMILY, EMPLOYMENT, AND SOCIAL STABILITY

Many follow-up studies of treated alcoholics show surprisingly little interest in social changes (e.g., Smith, 1959; Jensen and Ramsay, 1963). The effects of various treatments on social stability, employment status, family relationships, and residential mobility are rarely considered. This neglect is especially true of studies of LSD in the treatment of alcoholism. None of the LSD studies quoted earlier in this chapter assessed its effects on such variables. Several of them appear to have involved the collection of relevant data but they have apparently been left unanalyzed (e.g., MacLean *et al.*, 1961). Only Savage (1962) specifically mentions social stability in his follow-up; 63 per cent of his alcoholics treated with LSD claimed an improvement in "external events" such as income, abode, and occupation. It might be that data on social stability frequently enter into the judgments of "improved," "much improved," and "unimproved,' but the manner of construction of these categories is not clear. It seems, however, that changes in drinking behavior alone have been taken to be the sole or most important effect of LSD therapy. At present, it is uncertain whether LSD has effects important and extensive enough to create major changes in the performance of the social roles of alcoholics.

The neglect of the social criteria of successful therapy is surprising from several points of view. LSD treatment in almost all cases was not oriented solely to modifying drinking behavior. Changes in social and family relationships are almost invariably a part of the psychiatric treatment for alcoholics. Also, it might be that important effects of LSD treatment would be missed if drinking behavior alone was the criterion for success. It should also be realized that insight gained from LSD might be used in a number of ways other than solely to understand drinking behavior, e.g., to improve social, familial, and occupational relations. Even if insights about drinking behavior alone were achieved, radical improvements in drinking pathology should lead to increased social stability.

It could also be argued that the general and specific personality changes believed to result from LSD therapy would promote social stability. The expected effects of LSD in reducing anxiety and the attendant defense mechanisms should lead to less strained family and employment relationships. The expected changes in self-concept and greater self-acceptance could also lead to much improved social relationships with family members and work associates. It is unfortunate that investigations of these areas have not been part of the previous LSD studies with alcoholics, for they might repay careful study.

4. Methods of the A.R.F. Investigation

EMPIRICAL AND METHODOLOGICAL CONSIDERATIONS

AS DESCRIBED EARLIER, numerous clinical trials have been made with LSD in the treatment of alcoholism and the reports of these trials have claimed that it markedly reduces drinking among alcoholics. Despite the large number of clinical investigations made and the alleged beneficial effects of LSD, there is little *convincing* evidence for its efficacy with alcoholics. Previous LSD trials are characterized by a lack of the control groups, follow-up procedures, and measures of change which would warrant unambiguous conclusions. Similarly, the personality changes in alcoholics treated with LSD have been established not with reliable and valid psychological tests but by clinical judgments. Usually clinical judgments of personality are found to be much less accurate than actuarial ones based upon psychological tests (Meehl, 1954).

The A.R.F. study of LSD is concerned with the effects of a single LSD experience under controlled conditions on the behavior of alcoholics. Chief among these conditions are blind administration, the provision of untreated control groups, the conduct of routine follow-ups, and psychological test measurements to assess personality changes. In addition, several areas of behavior were investigated which have not previously been covered. The follow-up interviews were concerned with personality changes and with social, familial, and occupational functioning, as well as with drinking behavior. Although we feel the present study is a step forward in the study of LSD, it cannot be considered a scientific panacea for the investigation of all questions concerning the drug. It is hoped that it will add to our knowledge in this area, but many further studies with varying conditions and procedures will be necessary to fully understand its effects.

THE ALCOHOLIC PATIENTS AND THEIR ASSIGNMENT
TO TREATMENT GROUPS

There were 30 patients employed in this study; 28 were males and 2 were females. All were alcoholic in-patients or day-care patients at the Toronto Clinic of the Addiction Research Foundation. All had a long history of excessive and uncontrolled drinking, previous unsuccessful attempts at therapy, and only short periods of abstinence in the year prior to their appearance at the clinic. The average age of the patients was 40 years. These alcoholics presented a variety of psychiatric diagnoses, in addition to the basic diagnosis of chronic alcoholism. Thirteen were diagnosed as passive–aggressive personalities, eight as compulsive or obsessive personalities, two as chronic depressives, two as immature personalities, and one each as paranoid, cyclothymic, anxiety neurotic with depressive features, and pseudo-neurotic schizophrenic. There were no patients with a diagnosis of overt psychosis.

The patients used were volunteers "for the study of a new drug." Since many more patients volunteered than could be accommodated, the group of 30 which was chosen at random should represent the total in-patient and day-care population in terms of social and drinking characteristics. Some of those who volunteered were excluded because of major cardiac or hepatic disease, or because of incipient psychoses, any of which might have been worsened by LSD. Patients with previous psychoses or previous delirium tremens were not excluded. In addition, three patients who originally volunteered withdrew before the drugs had been given and hence their data have not been used.

The 30 alcoholics were divided into three groups of 10 each. The LSD group received a single 800 μg dose of LSD intramuscularly in a specially arranged session during their therapy. The Ephedrine group received a 60 mg dose of ephedrine sulphate made up to the same volume intramuscularly in a similar session. Both of these Drug groups were compared with a Control group which was exposed to all of the procedures and therapies given to the Drug groups except for the drug session. Ephedrine sulphate was used as a control drug for LSD because it is relatively innocuous, has no therapeutic use in alcoholism and no hallucinogenic effect, and because some of its effects—nervousness, headache, palpitations, nausea, and vertigo—could be confused with the earliest effects of LSD which are mainly physiological. It was expected, in view of the wide variety of responses to LSD, that the use of ephedrine might make it difficult for patients to determine that two different drugs were being used.

For each week in which there were volunteers the chief investigator (R.G.S.) selected one person at random from a list of volunteers. Each patient was then randomly assigned to a Drug or Control group according to a prearranged schedule. Patients assigned to the Drug group were further delegated to the LSD or Ephedrine group in a random order established by our statistical consultant.[6] Neither the investigators, nor personnel at the Toronto Western Hospital, nor clinic personnel at A.R.F. knew which patients in the Drug groups received LSD except as it became apparent during the treatment interview. However, in 19 out of 20 cases the LSD therapist guessed correctly which drug the patient had received. This was an unexpected finding as it was hoped that the ephedrine and LSD effects would be more similar. However, the LSD therapists did not give therapy beyond the post-treatment session and therapists at the A.R.F. clinic where the post-treatment therapy took place were completely "blind" as to which patients received LSD. In nearly every case the patient continued to believe that he had received a magical "new drug" even if he had actually received ephedrine sulphate. Case files and therapy records of all patients in the Drug groups were examined for indications that the blind control was not achieved, but the indications are that full blindness was achieved for the patient group.

The random assignment of patients to treatment groups appeared to be successful in equalizing the groups before the study began. For example, there were no significant differences between the groups in age or sex composition, education (completed years of school), marital status, occupation, or drinking pattern. Unfortunately, there were slightly but not significantly more alcoholics in the LSD group who were unemployed at the

[6]Special thanks are due to Dr. A. S. Phillips, Statistician, Canadian Cancer Society, for help in this regard.

time of their hospitalization. Fortunately, the numerous similarities provided considerable assurance that the groups were well matched for a number of characteristics known to affect success in therapy. As later analyses will show, the groups were also very similar in a number of drinking history variables.

THE TREATMENT SETTING

Because this study examines the effects of the addition of LSD to an existing treatment for alcoholism it is necessary to outline the treatment. A description of it has already been published (Gibbins and Armstrong, 1957) but a few details are relevant here. All patients are in-patients or day-care patients in a small hospital devoted to alcoholism and drug addiction. As a part of their therapy they attend a series of didactic meetings or group psychotherapy sessions concerned with problems of alcohol use, and with their motivations for excessive drug use. These sessions are held every morning and afternoon. In addition, physio- and occupational therapy facilities are available, together with opportunities for individual case work and psychiatric interviews. In many ways the approach is similar to that of the Yale Plan clinics, except that in-patient facilities are provided and certain concepts of therapeutic community have been introduced. This has resulted in greater patient participation in disciplinary and social functions, and in the breakdown of some of the traditional formalism of such clinics (Jones, 1952). The orientation of the professional staff is to see alcoholism as an illness that can be cured or alleviated by medical and psychiatric treatment and by the patient's efforts at total abstinence. After in-patient and day-care treatment, patients are encouraged to maintain out-patient or social-recreational contacts with the clinic.

EVALUATIONAL PROCEDURES BEFORE DRUG ADMINISTRATION

A number of psychological tests and questionnaires were administered to all patients to ensure their comparability before treatment and to provide a baseline from which to assess post-treatment improvements. Patients were given a battery of tests including the Maudsley Personality Inventory, the Haigh–Butler Q Sort, the Rorschach, and a shortened form of the Wechsler Adult Intelligence Scale. They were also interviewed as to their marital status, occupational history, education, and treatment experiences. In addition, a drinking questionnaire concerned with many facets of the patient's drinking in the past year was given. The questions related to period of abstinence, the number of drinking occasions and the amounts drunk on those occasions, the types of beverage used, and the occurrence of symptoms associated with alcoholism. All questions were constructed to yield definite quantifiable answers rather than general impressions. The complete questionnaire is given in Appendix A.

In addition to the tests and questionnaires, a detailed psychiatric examination was made by the LSD therapist prior to the drug experience. At this time efforts were made to establish rapport between the patient and the LSD therapist and to begin a therapeutic relationship which could be pursued during LSD treatment. A psychiatric diagnosis and prognosis was arrived at. All tests, questionnaires, and examinations were administered in a standardized form to all patients regardless of their treatment group.

ADMINISTRATION OF LSD AND EPHEDRINE

On the day the drug was given, the patients went to the psychiatric ward of a general hospital (Toronto Western) without breakfast. All had been off drugs for three days, except those who had been receiving dilantin sodium to prevent seizures. If patients were on this drug it was maintained and if not then a 250-mg dose was administered intramuscularly, as an anticonvulsant precaution, shortly after admission to the ward. Each patient was placed in a single room, attached to the bed by a light but strong (Posey) belt for security. Either 800 μg of LSD or 60 mg of ephedrine sulphate were administered intramuscularly according to a prearranged schedule. A particularly large dose of LSD was used in order to be certain that important effects were not missed by using minimal doses.

After the drug administration the patients were attended throughout a three-hour interview by a doctor and a nurse as co-therapists. The three-way psychotherapeutic interview attempted to (*a*) discover a meaningful alternative to the patients' habitual anesthetic use of alcohol, and (*b*) define the patients' attitudes in the following areas:

1. Transference feelings towards doctor and nurse
2. Displacement feelings towards the act of drinking
3. Child–parent relationship
4. Suicidal propensity
5. Displacement attitudes towards alcohol
6. Genital–sexual and urethral–sexual behavior
7. Co-ordination between verbal and non-verbal behavior.

All of the personnel administering the LSD therapy had had long acquaintance with it and had undergone the experience themselves. It is uncertain whether this is essential for best results as Smith's first study (1958) was done before he had taken LSD himself. Therapists at the Toronto A.R.F. clinic had had no personal experience with LSD.

After the drug wore off, each patient remained in his bed on the ward overnight, sedated with chlorpromazine if necessary, and released to the A.R.F. clinic on the next day. Patients in the Control group received all the tests and evaluations and had access to the same therapies but did not go to the Toronto Western Hospital or receive LSD or ephedrine. Thus, they received the same psychiatric and medical attention as those in the Drug groups, except for the drug administration.

Whatever insights or understandings were gained from the drug session were used by the patient in his individual or group psychotherapy meetings. A.R.F. therapists made no special effort to examine the results of the drug sessions unless the patient requested it. However, most patients who received LSD or ephedrine did work through the experience with their own therapists and also with other patients who received drugs. There was also a post-LSD therapeutic interview with the LSD therapist during which insight and feelings developed during the LSD or ephedrine session could be discussed and clarified. This interview was held about five days after the drug administration. Other than this post-treatment interview, however, responsibility for using the LSD experience in treatment rested with the A.R.F. therapists who afterwards discussed this experience with the patients.

POST-TREATMENT EVALUATION AND FOLLOW-UP

On the day after the drug session patients in the two drug groups returned to the A.R.F. clinic to complete their in-patient treatment. The average length of stay after the drug session was about one week.

All patients were exposed to the same follow-up procedures after their release from the clinic. The first follow-up was timed to occur six months after the initial evaluation. A two-week leeway was allowed around this six months ideal and special efforts were made to interview and retest patients within these limits. All of them were seen within eight months after their initial testing. Unlike many earlier studies on LSD the follow-up was completely successful in that all 30 patients were seen. During the follow-up, patients were contacted by the same research assistant so that interexaminer biases were controlled.[7] The same tests and drinking questionnaire used in the pre-treatment evaluation were administered during follow-up except that information on drinking was sought for the period since the last testing. Three patients died during the period covered by the study but all died after their first follow-up had been completed.

A second follow-up was begun two years after the beginning of the LSD study, or about 18 months after the end of the first follow-up.[8] During this follow-up it was found that patients were much more difficult to find because of greater occupational and

[7]The success of this follow-up was due primarily to the efforts of Richard Bennett who conducted all but one of the interviews.

[8]This follow-up was conducted by Mrs. M. Marley of the Addiction Research Foundation.

residential mobility. It was impossible to time this second follow-up so that all patients were seen during the same interval after their treatment. In addition, only 24 of the remaining 27 patients were interviewed, as the others had left the country and all efforts to contact them were unsuccessful. The second follow-up was concerned solely with drinking behavior and not with personality changes, so that only the drinking history questionnaire was administered.

PSYCHOLOGICAL TEST ADMINISTRATION

All alcoholics in the Drug groups received a battery of psychological tests a few days before their drug session, and those in the Control group had the battery at the same relative time in their hospital treatment. The same tests were administered as part of the first follow-up study which was made six months after their first testing. The Rorschach, Maudsley Personality Inventory, and Haigh-Butler Q Sort were administered on both occasions.

Maudsley Personality Inventory

The Maudsley Personality Inventory (M.P.I.) is a well-standardized questionnaire which yields independent measures of introversion and neuroticism based on factor analysis. The M.P.I. has usually shown high test–retest reliability (0.62 to 0.80). Its validity was established by its high correlations with other questionnaire measures of introversion and neuroticism (summarized by Eysenck, 1957) and with learning and perceptual measurements of these characteristics. A decrease in neuroticism from the pre-treatment to the post-treatment period was expected in the LSD group because of earlier claims that LSD reduces the need for inappropriate defense mechanisms such as repression, decreases self-consciousness, anxiety, and guilt, and promotes "tranquility." Any or all of these changes should be reflected in decreased neuroticism scores although the M.P.I. does not directly measure these separate personality features. No special expectations were entertained for changes in introversion–extroversion scores.

Rorschach

The Rorschach was administered as a standard projective test eliciting information about general personality functioning. The Rorschach was used essentially as a clinical technique rather than as an objective test. It was expected that the number of human movement responses (M) would increase in the LSD group since LSD is believed to loosen repression, increase sensitivity to others, and allow objective appraisals of the self. Human movement responses are usually taken to indicate the presence of such personality characteristics (Schafer, 1954). It was also expected that the number of responses (R) on the Rorschach would be greater, also indicating decreased repression (Schafer, 1954). Color responses (FC, CF, C) were expected to increase as evidence of increased sensitivity to others. Shading responses (K, FK) were expected to decrease as an indication that anxiety was reduced.

All Rorschachs were scored by the same clinical psychologist, according to the Klopfer system (Klopfer, Kelley, and Davidson, 1946). The scorer was unaware of which patients had received the various treatments and hence her scoring was a completely blind analysis.[9]

Some criticisms have been made of research which isolates and counts only a few determinants in Rorschach protocols. It has been argued that such determinants should not be considered separately but only as part of the whole record. Accordingly, an experienced clinical psychologist made ratings of change which appear in the post-treatment Rorschachs over those obtained in the pre-treatment period. The two Rorschachs for each patient were examined together when an over-all estimate was made of whether repression, anxiety, internal conflict, and guilt feelings were more, less, or equally evident in the post-treatment compared with the pre-treatment Rorschach. The same ratings were made of the range of emotion displayed, and the degree of self-acceptance indicated. Both the ratings and scoring were "blind" in that the rater did not know which treatment had been received by any patient.

[9]Special thanks are due to Mrs. Toby Levinson who scored and evaluated all of the Rorschach protocols.

Haigh–Butler Q Sort

The Haigh–Butler Q Sort was developed to assess changes in self-concepts which occur as a result of psychotherapy. The patient sorts 100 cards containing statements related to the self. These cards are sorted into eight piles according to a normal curve expressed as a scale from "least like me" to "most like me." Two sorts are made—a "self-sort," describing the patient as he is today, and an "ideal sort," describing him as he would like to be. Patients were given unlimited time. It has been found (Rogers and Dymond, 1954; Ends and Page, 1959) that correlations between self and ideal sorts are low before therapy, but much higher afterward. It has also been found (Rogers and Dymond, 1954) that those patients judged clinically to be most improved show the highest correlation between self and ideal sorts after therapy.

All alcoholics in this study did the Q sorts at the beginning of their hospital stay and six months after their release. Again, all test results were scored without knowledge of the treatments assigned to individual patients. It was expected that those in the LSD group would show greater correlations between self and ideal sorts after therapy than would the non-LSD groups. This expectation was based on the previous speculations that the therapeutic effects of LSD were marked by changes in self-concept, and by greater self-acceptance.

EFFECTIVENESS OF CONTROLS AND DOUBLE-BLIND PROCEDURES

The validity of a study such as this turns on the effectiveness of the control procedures and on the degree of blindness achieved. At the outset, it was hoped that none of the patients would be aware that LSD was being used and communications with them referred only to a "new drug" study. However, publicity in newspapers and other media convinced many patients that some hallucinogen was being administered, although this was not clarified by the clinical staff. Patients were not aware that *two drugs* were being used and they had no way of knowing which patients received LSD and which ephedrine. They were told that there is a great variation in how people react to the drug, that some react in a striking way and that some react only slightly. This appeared to create an effective blind condition so far as the patients were concerned. Patients who got ephedrine interpreted it as a slight reaction to LSD. Both staff and patients knew which patients were in the Control group and receiving no drug. Blindness was obtained in that patients and staff at A.R.F. were not aware of which drug was given in a particular instance although the LSD therapists guessed. Thus, although complete double-blindness was not achieved a modified single-blindness was.

Further efforts to control biases due to expectation or suggestion were associated with the conditions for follow-up and data analysis. The follow-up worker did not know, at any time, which patient had received which treatment. More precautions were taken to make a blind analysis of treatment outcome, in that all ratings, measurements, and final analyses were completed before the drug code was broken. That is, the data on drinking and abstinence were analyzed and interpreted as being differences between groups A, B, and C, with no knowledge of these designations until the study was completed.

5. Results of the A.R.F. Investigation

DRINKING BEHAVIOR

BECAUSE THE SAME INFORMATION about drinking was sought for the pre- and post-treatment periods, the major results are concerned with differences in drinking during these times. The first follow-up was conducted six months after treatment and the most detailed data are for this period. Table IV shows the age, sex, number of years at school, and employment for each patient at the time of entry into the clinic and it can be seen that there are no significant group differences in these variables. Table IV also shows the percentage gain in weeks of longest abstinence and the percentage gain in total weeks of abstinence. These figures were arrived at by expressing the number of weeks in the longest abstinence and in the total period of abstinence as a percentage of the total number of weeks in the pre- and post-treatment periods. The figures shown represent the gains made in the first post-treatment period over the pre-treatment period. Simple inspection indicates that there is a significant gain in abstinence for all three groups with average gains of 33.7 (LSD), 31.5 (Ephedrine), and 19.6 per cent (Control). However, simple analyses of variance showed that there are no differences between the LSD, Ephedrine, and Control groups in percentage gain in total abstinence ($F = 0.323$, $P > 0.05$) or in their longest period of abstinence ($F = 0.463$, $P > 0.05$).

Aside from increasing periods of abstinence it was felt that LSD might reduce the actual number of drinking occasions. Accordingly, the answers to the questions on the number of drinking occasions (parts II, III in the follow-up questionnaire) were analyzed for group differences. The average number of times per month the groups had one or more drinks in the pre-treatment period was 13.9 (LSD), 23.3 (Ephed.), and 19.4

70

TABLE IV

PATIENT CHARACTERISTICS AND THE PERCENTAGE GAIN IN ABSTINENCE IN THE POST-TREATMENT OVER THE PRE-TREATMENT PERIOD

Group	Patient number	Age	Sex	Marital status*	No. of yr. at school	Employed or unemployed	Psychiatric diagnosis	Gain in abstinence (%)
Control	1	43	M	D	15	U	Obsessive personality	69.2
	2	57	M	M	7	U	Chronic depression—borderline IQ	69.3
	3	29	M	Sep.	7	U	Passive—aggressive personality	-57.7
	4	40	M	S	17	E	Compulsive personality	100.0
	5	43	M	M	6	U	Compulsive personality—epilepsy	13.4
	6	37	M	S	17	E	Cyclothymic personality	-76.9
	7	42	M	D	16	U	Immature personality	11.6
	8	33	M	M	10	E	Immature personality	-7.7
	9	39	M	M	12	U	Passive—aggressive personality	63.5
	10	45	F	C.L.	8	Housewife	Chronic depressive state—borderline IQ	11.5
LSD	1	59	M	Sep.	12	E	Passive—aggressive personality	-11.5
	2	36	M	S	9	U	Passive—aggressive personality	63.5
	3	38	M	M	8	U	Passive—aggressive personality	90.4
	4	30	M	M	9	U	Passive—aggressive personality	7.7
	5	47	M	M	10	U	Psychoneurosis with anxiety and depression	7.7
	6	26	M	S	10.5	U	Paranoid personality	61.5
	7	27	M	S	17	U	Compulsive personality—organic brain syndrome	-5.8
	8	47	M	D	10	U	Pseudo-neurotic schizophrenia	59.7
	9	50	M	Sep.	11.5	U	Passive—aggressive personality	50.0
	10	31	F	Sep.	9	Housewife	Compulsive Personality (with depression)	13.5
Ephedrine	1	49	M	M	18	E	Passive—aggressive personality	34.6
	2	33	M	M	16	U	Passive—aggressive personality	63.5
	3	45	M	M	19	E	Paranoid personality	23.1
	4	44	M	M	10.5	E	Passive—aggressive personality	1.9
	5	37	M	Sep.	12	E	Passive—aggressive personality	7.7
	6	35	M	Sep.	6	E	Passive—dependent personality	50.0
	7	35	M	M	10	U	Obsessive—compulsive personality	53.8
	8	48	M	Sep.	16	U	Obsessive—compulsive personality	0.0
	9	38	M	C.L.	12	U	Passive—aggressive personality	3.9
	10	28	M	S	10	E	Compulsive personality (chronic anxiety state)	76.9

*D, Divorced; S, single; Sep., separated; M, married; C.L., common law.

(Cont.), and in the first post-treatment period the data showed no significant differences among the groups (Appendix B, Table I). This result shows that the three groups were well matched in extent of drinking in the pre-treatment period. The lack of group differences in the post-treatment period indicates no significant effect of LSD on the number of drinking occasions.

Results similar to those above were also obtained for the number of occasions per month on which the patients became drunk (Appendix A, question II, iv). Patients in the three groups became drunk on 5.5 (LSD), 2.6 (Ephedrine), and 11.1 (Control) occasions per month in the pre-treatment period and on 3.1, 2.5, and 3.4 occasions, respectively, in the first post-treatment period. A variance analysis on these data (Appendix B, Table II) showed a significant reduction in the number of drunkenness occasions in the post-treatment period for the three groups combined. But, again there were no differences between treatment groups and no differential effect of LSD.

The effects of the various treatments on a number of drinking symptoms were also investigated. These symptoms (Appendix A, question II, 5) cover such behavior as increasing preoccupation with drinking, neglecting meals, drinking only for the effect of alcohol, morning drinking, getting drunk on a working day, blackouts, and going on "binges." In order to assess changes in such behavior the numbers of patients answering "frequently," "sometimes," and "never" to each question were separately determined for the pre- and post-treatment periods. Changes from the pre- to the post-period were then recorded by counting the number of patients who reported that a behavior changed from frequently to sometimes or never, and from sometimes to never. Patients whose symptoms increased or remained the same were also counted. Chi-square analyses (2×3) were made to determine whether the three groups differed in that more patients in some groups experienced a reduction in symptoms. All of these analyses were non-significant in outcome. Hence LSD does not seem to reduce the reported frequency of the following symptoms —morning drinking, getting drunk on a working day, blackouts, being preoccupied with alcohol, neglecting meals, and drinking only for the effects of alcohol.

It was also thought that LSD, even if it did not directly reduce drinking or drunkenness, might facilitate therapy by helping patients to establish a closer contact with the clinic. Accordingly, the total number of contacts which each patient had with the clinic were counted for the pre- and post-treatments separately. The number of contacts for the pre-treatment period were 8.0, 6.0, and 6.7 for the LSD, Ephedrine, and Control groups respectively, and 5.6, 5.9, and 4.3 for the post-treatment period. Simple analyses of variance were made separately for the differences in the pre-treatment and the post-treatment periods. For both there were no significant differences ($F = 0.081$, $P > 0.05$ and $F = 0.135$, $P > 0.05$ respectively). This indicates that the groups were well balanced in terms of their pre-treatment involvement in therapy. It is also clear that LSD does not increase the alcoholic's involvement in therapy on the basis of frequency of therapeutic contact.

A further indication of changes in drinking problems was found in the court and prison appearances for each alcoholic. The groups each had three incarcerations during the one-year pre-test period; the Control and Ephedrine groups fell to one and two respectively in the post-treatment period but the LSD group remained at three. Convictions for drunkenness showed a somewhat different pattern (Appendix B, Table III) with the Control and Ephedrine groups both showing a drop from the pre- to the post-period (two to one and eight to four respectively). However the LSD group had more convictions in the first post-treatment period than in the pre-treatment (four to six). Convictions for impaired driving dropped from one in each group (pre-treatment) to none (post-treatment). These court and prison appearances substantiate the questionnaire data in that they indicate an over-all reduction in drinking and drunkenness but the data do not favor any particular group. The LSD group would seem to have slightly less change than the others in drinking if convictions for drunkenness alone are considered.

For most patients, collateral information on drinking in the post-treatment period was available from friends, relatives, or from their therapists. In all cases the correspondence with the patient's information was very good. Similar correlations reported by O'Reilly and Funk (1964) also lend support to the reliability of patient statements about their own abstinence.

An attempt was made to obtain a second follow-up interview with each patient. These follow-ups were planned to cover the period of one year to 18 months after the first follow-up. However, a number of occurrences made it impossible to conduct a complete and detailed follow-up on the second occasion. First of all, it was found that after 18 months the patients were very widely scattered. On the first follow-up all the patients were located in Ontario (most in Toronto); however on the second occasion some were as far away as Alberta, Baffin Island, Arizona, and Virginia. Interviews were difficult to obtain with these highly mobile and uncooperative alcoholics. Patients who had been in the Ephedrine group were the least cooperative and only six out of nine interviews could be obtained. Interviews with all other living patients were obtained. Three patients died before the second follow-up— two in the LSD group and one in the Ephedrine group. Two of these deaths were from natural causes associated with alcoholism (liver cirrhosis, and choking while intoxicated); the third was a suicide (barbiturate poisoning) and this involved one of the LSD patients. The role of the LSD experience in precipitating the suicide, if any, is unknown as the patient was far from the clinical facilities and had no close relatives in whom he confided. A close connection seems unlikely as the suicide occurred about one year after the LSD experience.

Follow-up information was obtained for drinking behavior and for social, occupational, and family relationships. The psychological tests were not given on the second occasion. More global judgments of change and improvement were made with the second set of follow-up data than with the first because of their incomplete nature.

Comparisons of the Ephedrine group with the LSD and Control groups are impossible because of the small number of interviews. Three patients in the Ephedrine group were seen 12 months after the first follow-up interview, and three 18 months after it. Three had been sober for at least 11 months with only a few short "benders," and two had maintained sobriety without strong cravings for alcohol and without the use of other drugs. Another

74

patient demonstrated heavy, uncontrolled drinking over the entire year with an average of five drunkenness occasions per week. Two more patients had shown slight improvement in drinking control but had been drinking heavily about half the time. Three patients could not be induced to participate. All of them seem to be drinking heavily from time to time but their geographic mobility and their hostility to the clinic make this difficult to clarify.

All ten patients in the Control group were interviewed and their reports have been supplemented with those of relatives and therapists. Only two had been completely abstinent since the first follow-up. Another patient had only a few short "benders" in his 14-month period since the first follow-up. Three more had been drinking constantly in an uncontrolled fashion—each for about 18 months, with little indication of a reduction of intake. The remaining four patients had been drinking during one-third to three-quarters of the weeks since the first follow-up and had retained considerable improvement in drinking control from their pre-treatment period. In summary, three patients were "much improved," four "somewhat improved," and three were "unimproved," in comparison with their pre-treatment drinking experiences.

The second follow-up interviews for the LSD group indicated less improvement than for the Control group. None of the eight living LSD patients was completely abstinent or even abstinent except for a few slips. One patient was drinking constantly during the one-year interval, and was frequently drunk. Three patients were drinking constantly in an uncontrolled manner for more than three-quarters of the follow-up interval. The other four patients showed an improvement in that drinking and drunkenness were common during about one-third to three-quarters of their follow-up periods. To summarize, none of the LSD patients was "much improved," three were "somewhat improved," and four were "very slightly improved," in comparison with their pre-treatment drinking behavior.

It should be noted that some patients in all three groups had improved markedly at the time of the first follow-up, including several in the LSD group. Attempts made by the LSD therapists to prognosticate improvement in drinking on the basis of information in the LSD interview proved no better than chance. However, in retrospect, three factors appear to differentiate the patients in the LSD group who gained in abstinence from those who did not. Under LSD, patients who *did not* gain in abstinence expressed ambivalent (love–hate) feelings toward the nurse, expressed suicidal wishes, and showed obvious lack of correlation between verbal and non-verbal behavior. Patients who *did* gain in abstinence expressed univalent (love or hate) feelings toward the nurse; all wanted to live and showed good correlation between verbal and non-verbal behavior. A further more extensive study would be required to confirm these tentative findings.

PSYCHOLOGICAL CHANGES

Results from the psychological tests are available for both the pre-treatment and the first post-treatment periods. All analyses are for differences among the three treatment groups in their pre- and post-treatment scores.

Maudsley Personality Inventory

The mean neuroticism and extroversion scores for the pre- and post-treatment testings are shown in Appendix B, Table IV. Analyses of the differences between means revealed no significant treatment effects ($F = 1.92$, and 0 respectively). LSD therapy had, then, no significant effect upon neuroticism or introversion.

On a more impressionistic level it could be argued that the neuroticism results show interesting trends. It might be noted here that all three groups show a decrease in neuroticism from the pre- to the post-treatment period. This decrease is greatest in the LSD group (mean difference = 7.8), less in the Control group, and least in the Ephedrine group. The results are at least in the direction expected, although the intergroup differences are not significant. These results would bear more extensive investigation in later studies of LSD.

Rorschach

The Rorschach was administered as a projective test of general personality functioning and also in order to test specific hypotheses about the effects of LSD. The hypotheses were that the LSD group would show more human movement responses (M), more color responses (FC, CF, C), and fewer shading responses (K).

The average number of M, C, and K in each group are shown in Appendix B, Table V. The number of shading responses (K) proved to be very small (less than one per group) and hence statistical analysis was impossible. On inspection, the number of shading responses does not seem to differ much from one group to another before or after treatment. However, there is a strong general trend towards fewer shading responses in the post-treatment as opposed to the pre-treatment period (27 compared to 12). This indicates at least some anxiety reduction as a result of the clinical treatment given, but no specific benefit from LSD therapy. Color (C) and human movement (M) responses were more numerous than shading. The frequencies of these responses are shown in Appendix B (Table V), with the total number of responses (R). Separate analyses for (C), (M), and (R) indicated no significant pre-treatment or post-treatment differences for any of the scores. From inspection of the means it can be seen that the Control group showed the largest increase in number of responses (R) and in number of human movement responses (M), whereas the LSD group did not change markedly in any Rorschach scores. No evidence has been found for a strong treatment effect on any Rorschach scores nor is there any evidence for an LSD effect on scores indicative of decreased anxiety, loosened repression, or increased sensitivity to others.

Statistical analyses of Rorschach protocols such as those mentioned are commonly made but are often criticized. If discrete responses are analyzed into particular scores, over-all clinical impressions and global judgments of personality functioning are lost. For these reasons the statistical analyses were supplemented by clinical judgments made by the psychologist who administered and scored most of the records. This psychologist was asked to compare the post-treatment with the pre-treatment Rorschach protocol and to look for global signs of decreased anxiety, repression, internal conflict, and guilt feelings. Judgments were also made about possible increases in the range of emotions displayed and the degree of self-acceptance.

Appendix B (Table VI) shows the judgments of Rorschach changes organized into the categories "same," "more," "less," and "uncertain" for each of the three groups. There are highly similar outcomes for the three groups. In general, it can be seen that patients remained the same in the range of emotions displayed and in the degree of self-acceptance achieved. Anxiety and guilt feelings are reduced in about half of the alcoholics in each group, but the reduction of internal conflicts and repressions varies between groups. The LSD group shows more loosening of repression and less internal conflict than does the Ephedrine group but it remains close to the Control group in both of these. None of these differences are statistically significant but they are sufficient to provoke further interest in LSD research. No clear benefits from LSD therapy were detected by clinical ratings of Rorschach changes.

Haigh–Butler Q Sort

The Q Sort yielded four distributions of item scores from each patient, pre-treatment self-sort, post-treatment self-sort, pre-treatment ideal sort, and post-treatment ideal sort. In addition, a criterion distribution (C–S) was taken from the study of self and ideal changes in psychotherapy by Ends and Page (1959). The C–S is "the mean pattern reflecting the highest degree of healthy psychological adjustment possible with the particular sample of statements used according to the statistically combined Q-sorts of five experienced clinical psychologists" (Ends and Page, 1959, p. 4). All ten possible correlations among these five sorts were calculated for each subject, and the correlation coefficients converted to Fisher's Zs.

The major dependent variables in this study were the *movement indices* (Ends and Page, 1959). Each of these indices is the difference between the mean Z for a treatment group between one pair of Q-sort distributions and the mean Z for another pair. The significance of the difference between mean Zs for a single group shows whether there was a change from the pre- to the post-treatment periods. The significance of the differences between groups on a given index shows whether there was differential change, depending upon the particular treatment. The indices used (which were those used by Ends and Page) and their interpretation is as follows:

(1) Post S–C–S *minus* Pre S–C–S (G minus D): tells whether the self tends to grow healthier or less healthy over the therapy or control period. Plus means adjustment increased.

(2) Post S–Post I *minus* Pre S–Pre I (F minus B): tells whether the self and ideal converged during the course of the therapy or control period. Plus means greater convergence.

(3) Pre I–Post I *minus* Pre S–Post S (H minus A): tells whether ideal or self changed more. Plus means the ideal was more stable.

(4) Post I–C–S *minus* Pre I–C–S (J minus I): tells whether the ideal tends to grow healthier or unhealthier during the course of the therapy or control period. Plus means ideal became healthier.

(5) Post S–Pre I *minus* Pre S–Pre I (E minus B): tells whether the self moved toward or away from the pre-ideal during the course of the treatment or control period. Plus means self moved toward pre-ideal.

(6) Post S–Post I *minus* Pre S–Post I (F minus C): tells whether the self moved toward or away from the post-ideal during the course of the therapy or control period. Plus means self moved toward the post-ideal.

(7) Pre S–Post I *minus* Pre S–Pre I (C minus B): tells whether the ideal tended to move toward or away from the pre-self during the therapy or control period. Plus means ideal moved toward the pre-self.

(8) Post S–Post I *minus* Post S–Pre I (F minus E): tells whether the ideal moved toward or away from the post-self during the therapy or control period.

t tests for correlated means were used to estimate the significance of each of these indices for a given group; *t* tests for uncorrelated means were used for the significance of differences on each index between treatment groups. All significance tests were two-tailed.

Appendix B (Table VI) shows the means, standard errors, and statistical outcomes for each of the eight *Q*-sort movements indices. Only one of the statistical tests out of the 24 performed is significant. The control groups showed a significant growth in the health of the ideal from the pre- to the post-treatment period. However, there are no over-all differences establishing the effectiveness of therapy on self or ideal sorts, nor are there indications that LSD is better, compared to either of the control treatments. Therapy as a whole then failed to (a) make the self grow healthier, (b) bring self and ideal closer together, (c) stabilize the ideal, (d) make the ideal healthier, (e) move the self toward the pre-ideal, (f) move the self toward the post-ideal, (g) move the ideal away from the pre-self, and (h) move the ideal toward the post-self. Any of these movements would have indicated progress in psychotherapy, and significant psychological changes during the post-treatment period.

As well as over-all analyses for each group separately, comparisons between groups were made for each of the movement indices. Again most of these were non-significant as can be seen from Appendix B (Table VIII). Four differences were significant at the rather lenient $P < 0.10$ level of significance. The LSD group gained significantly more than the Ephedrine group in healthiness of the self and in the movement of the self toward the post-ideal. The Controls showed greater convergence of self and ideal during therapy and also more movement of the self toward the post-ideal than did the Ephedrine group. All other differences were non-significant ($P > 0.10$).

More impressionistic analyses based on data in Appendix B (Tables IV, V, VI, VII, VIII) yield some additional results that are worthy of comment. The LSD group shows almost no change in the self-ideal discrepancy, whereas that discrepancy increases for the Ephedrine group. The ideal changed more in the LSD than in the Ephedrine group and also became healthier. Compared with the no-drug-control group, the self in the LSD became healthier and also the self and the ideal changed more in the LSD group. In a vague, and possibly unreliable manner, these results show some trends towards the changes predicted for alcoholics given LSD. However, they do not establish any important differences in the personality effects of the LSD, ephedrine, and control treatments.

80

The various treatments administered seemed to have little effect upon family relationships, and again the LSD therapy showed few benefits not achieved with other therapies. There were no over-all or group differences in numbers of patients living with their wives (Appendix B, Table IX), or in the degree of satisfaction felt in marital relationships. The reported frequency of marital fights or arguments showed few changes except for a slight over-all reduction in arguments about drinking. There were no indications that the alcoholic males were taking more family responsibilities in disciplining children or in handling household finances, but they seemed to be spending more time in social and recreational activities with their wives. Further, extramarital relationships showed a slight decrease in frequency during the first post-treatment period. None of these differences were more striking in the LSD group than in the others. Relationships with relatives (other than wives) and with neighbors and friends showed few quantitative or qualitative changes except for a decrease in the number of drinking occasions with friends.

All of the three groups showed relatively more residential mobility in the post-treatment period than in the pre-treatment period (Appendix B, Table X). There were no group differences in residential mobility.

Only one of the variables associated with employment showed any post-treatment change. The numbers of employed alcoholics were 4, 1, and 4 in the Control, LSD, and Ephedrine groups during the pre-treatment period, and 3, 5, and 4, respectively, during the post-treatment period. Only the alcoholics who got LSD made a substantial gain in employment. The three groups did not differ in average numbers of jobs held or in their feelings of satisfaction about those jobs.

Data from the second follow-up essentially parallel those of the first. There were no striking group differences in family or social relationships and again marked residential mobility occurred. A few more alcoholics in the LSD group than in the Control group were employed at the time of the second follow-up.

6. Discussion and Conclusions

DRINKING BEHAVIOR

THIS STUDY provides no evidence that LSD is a useful adjunct to psychiatric treatment for alcoholism. There is a remarkable consistency in the results for drinking, all of which point to "no effect." The LSD group did not differ from the other groups in gain in total abstinence, or in their longest period of abstinence, and they did not have fewer post-treatment occasions in which drinking or drunkenness occurred. Further, LSD does not seem to reduce or eliminate symptoms such as morning drinking, getting drunk on working days, blackouts, preoccupation with alcohol, neglect of meals, or drinking only for the effects of alcohol. Also, LSD did not reduce the number of convictions for drunkenness or for impaired driving. In addition, LSD does not seem to increase the alcoholic's involvement in therapy. The conclusion is that the LSD as administered had virtually no effect on the drinking of alcoholics.

These findings would seem to conflict with those found in earlier studies which assert that LSD is an effective adjunct to the treatment of alcoholism. Investigators such as Chwelos *et al.* (1959), Smith (1958), and MacLean *et al.* (1961) reported that LSD administration resulted in 50 to 94 per cent of their patients being "improved" or "much improved" at the time of follow-up. However, much of the contrast between the present findings and earlier ones is more apparent than real. All of the earlier investigators examined LSD as an adjunct to some other form of therapy such as group psychotherapy (MacLean *et al.*, 1961) or psychiatric treatment (Smith, 1958) just as was done here. The results of the present study, in a way, *confirm* these earlier reports in that eight out of ten patients could, after six months, be listed as "improved" or "much improved" in terms of increased abstinence and decreased drunkenness. However, in the present case, the improvement cannot be attributed solely to the use of LSD as the Ephedrine and Control groups showed comparable improvement. The important factor is that the earlier studies failed to use any non-LSD control groups against which the effects of LSD could be compared. If the earlier findings of an important LSD effect were due solely to the lack of controls, it would not be the first time in which controlled studies have shown effects very different from those of uncontrolled studies. For example, Glick and Margolis (1962), after a review of the literature on chlorpromazine, found that double-blind controlled studies yielded significantly fewer positive results than did non-blind, uncontrolled studies. In addition, studies by Griener (1950) indicate that khellin, a drug for angina pectoris, showed better effects than placebos in single-blind trials but results similar to placebos in double-blind trials.

The present study examined the effects of LSD under a specified set of conditions, and it cannot be argued that it answers all relevant questions about the drug. In this study as in any study there are a number of shortcomings and biases which, it might be thought, could lead to spuriously poor results. One of these is the small number of patients used—only ten in each group. However, earlier estimates of the effectiveness of LSD were sufficiently striking that ten cases should have demonstrated them. An added consideration is that studies involving follow-up are costly, time consuming, and difficult to execute. The procedural difficulties in following a large number of geographically mobile alcoholics are difficult to imagine for anyone who has not done so. Consequently the use of large numbers of patients has often resulted in less intensive work and hence in faulty data. For example, in Jensen and Ramsay's (1963) study of LSD large numbers of patients were used (N = 70 and 55 in LSD and Control groups), but almost 50 per cent of the patients in the Control group were lost to follow-up. The position is taken here that a controlled study with a small number of carefully studied patients is preferable to one that is loosely controlled and less intensive. There can be no doubt, however, that a controlled study with larger patient groups would be desirable.

It could also be argued that a *series* of LSD treatments is necessary with this particular group of alcoholics. However earlier studies (Chwelos *et al.*, 1959; Smith, 1958) reported beneficial effects with only one LSD experience.

Unexpected results with LSD might also have been obtained because of a myriad of details associated with the personnel and facilities involved. An impression gained from some earlier reports is that some trials were carried out by personnel committed to a belief in the value of LSD, or at least convinced that earlier papers had demonstrated some limited value. On the other hand, there was more neutrality about the value of LSD among the present investigators and no one was committed to a belief in its value, although all the investigators would have preferred to find that LSD was an effective therapy. The role of therapists' conviction and personal commitment to a treatment approach has rarely been investigated as a factor in its success but it might well be an important influence.

There are also questions concerning the role of various methods of LSD administration. It might be argued that the LSD procedures used here were different from those employed elsewhere and in some ways they were. Some workers (Chwelos *et al.*, 1959) have used music, visual stimuli such as pictures of relatives, cut flowers, and lists of questions about personal problems during the LSD session. None of these were used in the present study. Their importance in LSD therapy has never been assessed but they might well be vital elements in the patients' experience. Numerous other procedural details might also be crucially important to the LSD effect found in earlier studies, but they would require controlled evaluation to establish their importance. As we have noted LSD therapy was *just as effective here as in earlier studies,* with eight out of ten patients improved or much improved; however it was not more effective than treatment without LSD. Whether the refinements used by Chwelos *et al.* would have raised the improvement rate even higher than eight out of ten is uncertain and a matter for further experimentation. In a manner of speaking, then, therapy with LSD was effective here but it was *not more* effective than therapy without LSD. Accordingly, there is no compelling need to explain away the results obtained with LSD as they are similar to those obtained elsewhere.

The reader might also wonder whether the A.R.F. therapy was so effective prior to LSD that its addition could *not* improve upon this therapy. This is not the case as post-treatment changes could have been improved upon in almost all behaviors examined —drinking, drunkenness, personality, and social stability—in all but one or two patients in each of the groups. An earlier study of therapy at this clinic (Gibbins and Armstrong, 1957) reported that patients made an average gain in months of abstinence of only 36.3 per cent without LSD. Theoretically, therefore, its addition could have created a striking improvement in the effectiveness of the therapy offered.

Ideal conditions for a double-blind study of LSD were hoped for but not achieved. The similarities between LSD and ephedrine sulphate, although sufficient to confuse the patients, were not close enough to blind the therapists. More preliminary work might have been devoted to a search for a better control drug for LSD. It should also be remembered that patients correctly surmised that the "new drug" study was really a study of LSD. This probably created expectations of great benefit to be derived from participation in the drug groups. However, the net effects appear to be slight as the Control group—all of whom knew that they did not get the drug—did no worse than the Drug groups. Later studies should attempt to maintain secrecy about the identity of the drug being tested or at least provide some comparison between groups that are aware and not aware of what they are getting.

Regardless of these shortcomings, the present study has provided a no-drug control and a drug control group against which LSD can be evaluated. Further investigations examining the importance of each shortcoming could improve on the types of controls provided but could not dispense with them altogether.

Two additional controlled studies of LSD in the treatment of alcoholism have been made, but both are in the earliest stages of reporting. They confirm the present findings of "no effect" even though they used rather different doses of LSD, different clinical and evaluative procedures, and a variety of control groups. As yet, these studies have not been published in full detail but their broad outlines are obvious from preliminary reports.

A controlled study of LSD by Van Dusen *et al.* (1966) has appeared as a prepublication abstract. In this study 71 female alcoholics were given 400 μg of LSD, either singly or in groups of two to four. The sessions were held in a "pleasant private room with comfortable chairs and concert music." Forty-four patients received one session with LSD, 18 received two, and 9 received three. These patients were compared with a control group of 37 women who received the same therapy without LSD. Both groups were followed up after 6, 12, and 18 months. At the time of follow-up the two groups did not differ in abstinence, work history, social life, or social relations. Surprisingly, there were also no differences between the groups which received one, two, and three LSD sessions.

A preliminary report of a controlled LSD study has also been made by Johnson (1966). In Johnson's study 95 alcoholic clinic patients were randomly assigned to one of four groups: one group received one or two LSD sessions with concurrent psychotherapy, another received one or two LSD sessions with no psychotherapy, a third received a combination of sodium amytal and Methedrine with concurrent psychotherapy, and the last received only routine clinical care, with no drugs. Preliminary analyses of the follow-up data for one year indicate no difference in abstinence among the groups. All patients have not been followed up as yet and complete results will not be available until late in 1967.

It can be seen that both of these investigations appear to support the conclusion drawn from the present study, namely, that the evidence of a controlled evaluation does not support the view that LSD is a useful adjunct to the treatment of alcoholism. The rather different clinical procedures, LSD dosages, and control groups employed, lend additional weight to this conclusion, and tend to establish its generality in a way that a single study could never adequately accomplish.

PSYCHOLOGICAL CHANGES

An important aspect of LSD therapy in alcoholism has always been the claim that it provokes important psychological changes. In general, the effects are thought to be an uncovering of the unconscious, integration of ego functions, and a complete reordering of the emotional life. The psychological changes peculiar to alcoholism are supposed to be reductions in anxiety, guilt and repression, and the creation of the capacity to experience a wide range of emotions and to recognize conflicts more easily. However, the crux of the LSD transformation is thought to be increased self-acceptance. For example, Chwelos, *et al.* (1959) state that the "root of the therapeutic value of the LSD experience is its potential for producing self-acceptance." Most of these expectations, as with those concerned with drinking, are based upon uncontrolled studies with no pre- and post-LSD comparisons.

None of the expectations about psychological changes were clearly confirmed, although some suggestive trends can be noted. For example, neuroticism did not show a significantly greater decrease in the LSD group. However, in absolute terms the LSD group decreased more than the other two. Similar statements can be made about the Rorschach data. In general, they showed no significant statistical differences indicating greater anxiety reduction, loosened repression, or increased sensitivity to others. Nor did the clinical ratings of Rorschach change indicators favor the LSD group. On the other hand, more impressionistic analysis shows some trends towards greater psychological gains in the LSD group. Thus, it seems that the latter group showed a slightly wider range of emotions and less repression in the post-treatment period. However, there are indications of more anxiety, and internal conflict in those given LSD. It may be that a 6-month follow-up period is too short a time in which to evaluate changes and that the presumed deficits represent some sort of "working through" process. The stability and significance of these differences should be examined in larger studies with long-term follow-ups. At present, they can only be suggestive of further areas for research.

The results for the Q-Sort data on self and ideal concepts were also non-significant. It has been stated in several earlier papers that LSD promotes self-acceptance, but evidence for that assertion has not been found here. In fact, only the Control group showed significant growth in the health of ideal concepts from the pre- to the post-treatment period. Therapy, as a whole, did not affect the movement indices indicating that the self or ideal grew stronger after therapy; however, on two out of the three correlations reflecting adjustment before treatment the Ephedrine group is highest; on the other the LSD group is highest. After treatment, LSD is highest on all three, and the Ephedrine group lowest on two out of three. This provides some indication that the LSD group showed greater movement than the Ephedrine group, while the Control group remained steady. The LSD group showed the greatest increase in health of self-concept; in the Ephedrine group self-concept deteriorates after therapy. However, the Control group showed the greatest decrease in self-ideal discrepancy, and the greatest increase in the health of the ideal.

Several hypotheses can be deduced from these impressions. Perhaps standard clinical treatment affects the "ideal" self, but LSD moves the self-concept in a therapeutic direction. It seems that ephedrine treatment interferes with the movement of self and ideal concepts by creating anxiety or disappointment around the ephedrine injection with no therapeutic outcome. These possibilities provide a variety of avenues for further research on LSD effects on self-concept.

FAMILY RELATIONSHIPS, EMPLOYMENT, AND SOCIAL STABILITY

As with drinking behavior and personality few changes in social stability favored the LSD group. They did not differ from the others in a variety of marital behaviors or in the extent or quality of their relations with relatives and neighbors. Along with the other groups they showed a tendency to have fewer arguments about drinking and to spend more time with their families. However, the LSD group showed a striking improvement in the number of patients employed in the post-treatment period. This provides some evidence that it can affect variables related to social stability.

CONCLUSIONS

1. The present study was sufficiently related to earlier therapeutic trials with LSD in relevant details and in outcome to be considered a fair trial for the drug.

2. The results as a whole fail to indicate that the LSD experience *as described here* is an effective adjunct to the clinical treatment of alcoholism. Over-all improvements in drinking behaviors were found as a result of treatment, but these could not be attributed to the use of LSD.

3. LSD had no significant effects on the personality variables studied; however, there were indications that it promotes some therapeutic changes in self-concept.

4. LSD had no significant effects on social stability, except that more alchoholics given LSD were employed after therapy than in the control groups.

5. Earlier reports that LSD was an effective adjunct to therapy for alcoholism may have resulted from lack of adequate controls in the evaluation of its utility.

6. Further experimentation on various aspects of the LSD experience would be valuable, especially those concerned with personality variables.

7. Direction of Future Research
with LSD

SO FAR there has been a surfeit of research on various physical and psychological effects of LSD as well as a lack of scientific interest in the various treatment possibilities opened up by its use. The drug still seems to have a novelty value for investigators who continue to produce report after report about the most obvious and best understood effects of LSD (e.g., Kuramochi and Takahashi, 1964). Unfortunately, much of the clinical research on LSD is of questionable value and tends to give the impression that it was hastily carried out with few of the relevant theoretical or empirical questions answered or even formulated. The whole area of hallucinogenic drug exploration could benefit from studies of the basic parameters of the LSD reaction and from an elucidation of the importance of these parameters in treatment. All of these considerations have a special application to the use of LSD in the treatment of alcoholism. In this area there is an especially urgent need to investigate its crucial aspects as a therapy. An attempt will be made to suggest a few areas where research could be profitably pursued, for both a basic understanding of LSD and a greater appreciation of its potential role as a therapeutic agent with alcoholics. The most important of these relate to dosage, number of administrations, and the type of experience created by LSD.

There has been little consideration of the role of multiple doses of LSD in the treatment of alcoholism. The study reported here used only one dose and it is possible that a long series of administrations would have provoked more change. However, only one dose was used by several earlier investigators (Smith, 1959; MacLean *et al.*, 1961), who reported high rates of improvement. Other investigators have used several doses but the rationale for the selection of doses has never been made clear (Eisner and Cohen, 1958; Chandler and Hartman, 1960). If LSD achieved its maximum beneficial effects with a single dose it would be unique among the psychotherapeutic agents now available. Van Dusen *et al.* (1966) found that there was no difference in the abstinence or social stability scores of alcoholics given one, two, or three doses of LSD. An impressionistic look at Smith's data (Smith, 1959) suggests at least that those with multiple doses do no worse. It is possible, too, that in Smith's study only patients refractory to the first LSD experience were given multiple doses. More investigations in which various numbers of doses are compared for their effects, particularly a large series of doses, would settle this problem.

Another hiatus in our current knowledge concerns the minimal, maximal, and optimal doses for alcoholics. The dose used in the present study was 800 μg, which is somewhat higher than the doses used by Smith (200–400 μg), Chwelos *et al.* (200–400 μg), O'Reilly and Funk (200 μg), and Jensen and Ramsay (200 μg). Only MacLean *et al.* used doses as large as 800 μg and they varied their dosages from 400 to 1500 μg. Only the most impressionistic evidence is available on the therapeutic effects of high as opposed to low doses (200 μg). Studies comparing the therapeutic outcome of various doses with alcoholics have not been performed. However, the large doses used by McLean *et al.* (1961) and in the present study produced higher recovery rates than the low doses used by others.

Some controversy still exists about the optimal doses for alcoholics. An opinion has been expressed (MacLean *et al.*, 1961) that "small-dose techniques are less effective as they do not lead to a full realization of the therapeutic potential of the experience. Small doses do not alter the habitual frames of reference which may initially have induced the patient's problems, and often, reinforce those same unfavourable patterns of thinking and feeling which constitute his problems." A contrary opinion has been expressed (Jensen and Ramsay, 1963) that high doses (>200 μg) "do not result in more therapeutic effects. The resulting confusion or amnesia is undesirable and sometimes even disturbing to the patient when later, he is trying to establish for himself the reality of the experience." This latter position has not been borne out by published experiences with alcoholics, and dose–response studies are definitely required, at least with alcoholics.

Questions have also been raised about the type of therapeutic milieu that makes the best use of LSD. It is not known whether the therapist should take the drug at the same time as the patient as suggested by MacLean *et al.* (1961). There are also uncertainties about the necessity of the LSD therapist having himself had prior experience with the drug. For example, Smith (1958) believes that "the contact between therapist and patient can be improved if the therapist has taken the drug himself." However, Smith did not take LSD until the first series of sessions had been completed. The second series of alcoholics given LSD showed considerably higher improvement rates (15 out of 16 as opposed to 12 out of 24), although many other factors could also have been involved. In the present study those administering the LSD had considerable personal experience with it, but the clinic therapists had no direct experience at all. However, improvement rates with these naïve therapists were not much different from those obtained by therapists with LSD experience. Some investigations of the importance of the therapist's own experience with LSD would clarify and extend these conjectures.

Efforts should also be made to evaluate the importance of stimuli such as music, pictures of relatives, and of various therapeutic interventions during LSD. These techniques have been claimed to be useful and therapeutic by various investigators (Chwelos *et al.*, 1959; Smith, 1959), although they have not been systematically evaluated.

Surprisingly little attention has been paid so far to the types of alcoholic which can profit most and least from the LSD experience. There are indications that psychopaths and psychotics are least affected by LSD therapy (Smith 1958), but these studies are uncontrolled and such patients might be the most difficult to treat with any therapy. More investigations of the effects of LSD and control therapies on homogeneous groups of alcoholics are required before an estimate of the patients most likely to benefit from this experience can be defined. At present, those most likely to benefit from the drug would appear to be patients with essentially neurotic problems in addition to their alcoholism. There are no studies, as yet, of the effects of LSD on chronic drunkenness offenders—a group containing relatively small proportions of psychopathic personalities and psychotics. The remarkably strong LSD experience might conceivably provide sudden insights that would be difficult to provide for these alcoholics with conventional psychotherapy. Studies of LSD therapies with a wider variety of alcoholics than the usual middle class type found in clinics should be attempted.

It is also clear that LSD has generally been used as an adjunct to extensive psychotherapy, at least in the treatment of alcoholics. Various types of brief psychotherapy programs should be evaluated since there is no clear indication that LSD is of value only in lengthy therapies.

As yet, there have been few basic investigations of the mechanisms of LSD action in alcoholics. One should be able to identify the primarily emotional or broadly psychological factors in the LSD experience. There have been very few examinations of the acute psychological effects of LSD with alcoholics and even fewer long-term studies. The early assumption that it primarily modifies self-concepts does not seem to be borne out by the present results. In fact they suggest that LSD affects ideal concepts to a greater extent than self-concepts. Further studies of acute and long-term effects of LSD on psychological mechanisms should be made.

Questions have also been raised (Johnson, 1964) about the therapeutic effectiveness of LSD as a drug, when separated from other types of therapy. The abreactive and transcendental experiences triggered by LSD might be sufficient in themselves to create major behavioral changes, without the addition of individual or group psychotherapies. Some studies addressed to this problem are under way (Johnson, 1964). If the LSD experience itself is sufficient, then questions are raised about the need for LSD, since abreactions can be produced by other drugs with fewer side effects, for example, sodium amytal.

All of these questions deserve further controlled investigation, especially the possibility that less dangerous drugs than LSD could provide many of its important effects.

References

ABRAMSON, H. A. (ed.): The Use of LSD in Psychotherapy. New York, Josiah Macy Jr. Foundation, 1960.

ABRAMSON, H. A., JARVIK, M. E., & HIRSCH, M. W.: Lysergic acid diethylamide (LSD-25). X: Effect on reaction-time to auditory and visual stimuli, J. Psychol., 40, 39–52, 1955.

ABRAMSON, H. A., JARVIK, M. E., HIRSCH, M. W., & EWALD, A. T.: Lysergic acid diethylamide (LSD-25). V: Effect on spatial relations abilities, J. Psychol., 39, 435–42, 1955.

ABRAMSON, H., JARVIK, M., KAUFMAN, M., KORNETSKY, C., LEVINE, A., & WAGNER, M.: Lysergic acid diethylamide (LSD-25). I: Physiological and perceptual responses, J. Psychol., 39, 3–60, 1955.

ABRAMSON, H., JARVIK, M., LEVINE, A., KAUFMAN, M. R., & HIRSCH, M.: Lysergic acid diethylamide (LSD-25). XV: The effects produced by substitution of a tap water placebo, J. Psychol., 39, 367–83, 1955.

ARENDSEN-HEIN, G. W.: Hallucinogenic drugs: Specific problems, Lancet, 1, 445, 1961.

ARONSON, H., & KLEE, G. D.: Effect of lysergic acid diethylamide (LSD-25) on impulse control, J. Nerv. & Ment. Dis., 131, 536–9, 1960.

ARONSON, H., SILVERSTEIN, A. B., & KLEE, G. W.: Influence of lysergic acid diethylamide (LSD-25) on subjective time, A.M.A. Arch. Gen. Psychiat., 1, 469–72, 1959.

BACON, S. D.: State programs on alcoholism—a critical review. Fourteenth Annual Meeting, North American Association of Alcoholism Programs, 1963.

BAKER, E. F. W.: The use of lysergic acid diethylamide (LSD) in psychotherapy, Canad. M.A.J., 91, 1200–2, 1964.

BALDWIN, M., LEWIS, S. A., & BACH, S. A.: The effect of lysergic acid after cerebral ablation, Neurology, 9, 469–74, 1959.

BALL, J. R., & ARMSTRONG, J. J.: The use of LSD-25 (d-lysergic acid diethylamide) in the treatment of sexual perversions. Canad. Psychiat. A. J., 6, 231–5, 1961.

BENDA, P., & ORSINI, F.: Etude expérimentale de l'estimation du temps sous LSD-25, Ann. méd-psychol., 117, 550–7, 1959.

BENDER, L., FARETRA, G., & COBRINI, R. L.: LSD and UML treatment of hospitalized disturbed children, In Recent Advances in Biological Psychiatry, 5. New York, Plenum Press, 1963.

BENEDETTI, G.: Beispiel einer strukturanalytischen und pharmakodynamischen Untersuchung an einem Fall von Alkoholhalluzinose, Charakterneurose und psychoreaktiver Halluzinose, Ztschr. Psychotherap., u. med. Psychol. 1, 177–92, 1951. (Abst. in Annotated Bibliography, Delysid. Hanover, N.J., Sandoz Pharmaceuticals, 1958).

BERCEL, N. A., TRAVIS, L. E., OLINGER, L. B., & DREIKURS, E.: Model psychoses induced by LSD-25 in normals, Arch. Neurol. & Psychiat., 75, 588–618, 1956.

BLOUGH, D. S.: Effects of drugs on visually controlled behavior in pigeons, In Psychotropic Drugs, ed. by S. Garattini & V. Ghetti. New York, Elsevier, 1957.

BOARDMAN, W. K., GOLDSTONE, S., & LHAMON, W. T.: Effects of lysergic acid diethylamide (LSD) on the time sense of normals: A Preliminary Report, Arch. Neurol. & Psychiat., 78, 321–4, 1957.

BREHM, J. W., & COHEN, A. R.: Explorations in Cognitive Dissonance. New York, Wiley, 1962.

BUNNELL, S.: Chemistry and pharmacology of hallucinogenic drugs. Paper given at the LSD Conference, San Francisco, 1966.

Bureau on Alcoholism: Apparent results of referrals of alcoholics for LSD therapy (Interim Report), Saskatchewan Dept. Health and Welfare, Regina, Dec. 31, 1962.

Bureau on Alcoholism: Alcoholism Bulletin, Saskatchewan Dept. Health and Welfare, Regina, Feb., 1963.

BUSCH, A. K., & JOHNSON, W. C.: LSD-25 as an aid in psychotherapy, Dis. Nerv. System, 11, 241–3, 1950.

BUTTERWORTH, A. T.: Some aspects of an office practice utilizing LSD-25, Psychiatric Quart., 36, 734–53, 1962.

CARLSON, V. R.: Effect of lysergic acid diethylamide (LSD-25) on the absolute visual threshold, J. Comp. & Physiol. Psychol., 51, 528–31, 1958.

CHANDLER, A. & HARTMAN, M.: Lysergic acid diethylamide (LSD-25) as a facilitating agent in psychotherapy, A.M.A. Arch. Gen. Psychiat., 2, 286–99, 1960.

CHWELOS, N., BLEWETT, D. B., SMITH, C. M., & HOFFER, A.: Use of d-lysergic acid diethylamide in the treatment of alcoholism, Quart. J. Stud. Alcohol, 20, 577–90, 1959.

COHEN, S.: The Beyond Within: The LSD story. New York, Atheneum, 1964.

——— LSD: Problems and promise. Paper given at the LSD Conference, San Francisco, 1966.

COHEN, S., & DITMAN, K. S.: Complications associated with lysergic acid diethylamide (LSD-25), J.A.M.A. 181, 161–2, 1962.

——— Prolonged adverse reactions to lysergic acid diethylamide, Arch. Gen. Psychiat., 8, 475–80, 1963.

COHEN, S., FICHMAN, L., & EISNER, B. G.: Subjective reports of lysergic acid experiences in a context of psychological test performance, Am. J. Psychiat., 116, 30–5, 1958.

DITMAN, K.: Adverse reactions to hallucinogens. Paper given at the Conference on Drug Takers, Los Angeles, 1966.

DITMAN, K. S., HAYMAN, M., & WHITTLESEY, J.: Nature and frequency of claims following LSD, J. Nerv. & Ment. Dis., 134, 346–52, 1962.

DITMAN, K. W., & WHITTLESEY, J. R. B.: Comparison of the LSD-25 experience and delirium tremens, Arch. Gen. Psychiat., 1, 47–57, 1959.

EISNER, B. G., & COHEN, S.: Psychotherapy with lysergic acid diethylamide. J. Nerv. & Ment. Dis., 127, 528–39, 1958.

ENDS, E. J., & PAGE, C. W.: Group psychotherapy and concomitant psychological change, Psychol. Monogr., 73 (whole # 480), 1959.

EYSENCK, H. J.: The Dynamics of Anxiety and Hysteria. London, Routledge and Kegan Paul, 1957.

——— The effects of psychotherapy, In Handbook of Abnormal Psychology, edited by H. J. Eysenck, New York, Basic Books, 1960.

——— The effects of psychotherapy, In Handbook of Abnormal Psychology, edited by H. J. Eysenck, New York, Basic Books, 1961.

FESTINGER, L.: A Theory of Cognitive Dissonance. Evanston, Ill., Row, Peterson, 1957.

FONTANA, A. E.: El uso clinico de las drogas alucinogenas, Acta neuropsiquiat. Argent., 7, 94–8, 1961.

FOULDS, G.: Clinical research in psychiatry, J. Ment. Sc., 104, 259–65, 1958.

FREEDMAN, D. X.: Psychotomimetic drugs and brain biogenic amines, Am. J. Psychiat., 119, 843–50, 1963.

GIBBINS, R. J., & ARMSTRONG, J. D.: Effects of clinical treatment on behavior of alcoholic patients. Quart. J. Stud. Alcohol, 18, 429–50, 1957.

GIBERTI, F., GREGORETTI, L., & BOERI, G.: L'impiego della dietilamide dell'acido lisergico nells psiconervosi, Sistema nerv., 8, 191–208, 1956.

GLICK, B., & MARGOLIS, R.: A study of the influence of experimental design on clinical outcome in drug research, Am. J. Psychiat., 118, 1087–96, 1962.

GRIENER, T.: A method for the evaluation of the effects of drugs on cardiac pain in patients in angina of effort (A study of khellin (Visammin)). Am. J. Med., 9, 143–55, 1950.

HAAS, M., FINK, H., & HARTFELDER, G.: Das Placebo-problem. Fortschr. Arznei-mittelforsch., 1, 279–454, 1959. Trans. in Psychopharmacol. Service Center Bull. 8, 1–65, 1963.

HARTMAN, A. M., & HOLLISTER, L. E.: Effect of mescaline, lysergic acid diethyl-amide, and psilocybin on color perception. Psychopharmacologia, 4, 441–51, 1963.

HOFFER, A.: D-lysergic acid diethylamide (LSD): A review of its present status, Clin. Pharmacol. & Therapeutics, 6, 183–255, 1965.

HOFFER, A., OSMOND, H., & SMYTHIES, J.: Schizophrenia: A new approach. II: Result of a year's research, J. Ment. Sc., 100, 29–45, 1954.

HONIGFELD, G.: Temporal effects of LSD-25 and epinephrine on verbal behaviour. J. Abnorm. Psychol., 70 #4, Aug., 1965. Newsletter for research in Psychology, 6, 15–17, 1964.

ISBELL, H.: Comparison of the reactions induced by psilocybin and LSD-25 in man, Psychopharmacologia, 1, 29–38, 1959.

JARVIK, M. E., ABRAMSON, H. A., & HIRSCH, M. W.: Lysergic acid diethylamide (LSD-25). VI: Effect upon recall and recognition of various stimuli. J. Psychol., 39, 443–54, 1955.

JARVIK, M. E., ABRAMSON, H. A., HIRSCH, M. W., & EWALD, A. T.; Lysergic acid diethylamide (LSD-23). VIII: Effect on arithmetic test performance, J. Psychol., 39, 465–73, 1955.

JENSEN, S. E., & RAMSAY, R.: Treatment of chronic alcoholism with lysergic acid diethylamide, Canad. Psychiat. A. J., 8, 182–8, 1963.

JOHNSON, G. H.: Proposal to evaluate the use of LSD in the psychotherapy of alcoholism. Report of Medical Advisory Board, 1964. London Branch, Addiction Research Foundation, Toronto.

—— LSD research study—London Branch. Report to Professional Advisory Board, 1966. Alcoholism and Drug Addiction Research Foundation, Toronto.

JONES, MAXWELL: Social Psychiatry: A Study of Therapeutic Communities. London, Tavistock, 1952.

JOYCE, C. Experiments with control substances, Ann. Rheum. Dis., 20, 78–82, 1961.

KEY, B. J.: Effect of lysergic acid diethylamide on potentials evoked in the specific sensory pathways, Brit. M. Bull., 21, 30–5, 1965a.

—— The effects of drugs in relation to the afferent collateral system of the brain-stem, Electroencephalog. & Clin. Neurophysiol., 18, 670–9, 1965b.

KILLAM, K. F., & KILLAM, E. K.: (Abst.) The action of lysergic acid diethylamide on central afferent and limbic pathways in the cat, J. Pharmacol. & Exper. Therap. 166, 35, 1956.

KLOPFER, B., KELLEY, D. M., & DAVIDSON, H. H.: The Rorschach Technique. Yonkers, New York, World Book Co., 1946.

KNOWLES, J., & LUCAS, C.: Experimental studies of the placebo response, J. Ment. Sc., 106, 231–40, 1960.

KNUDSEN, K.: Homicide after treatment with lysergic acid diethylamide, Acta psychiat. scandinav., **180**, 389–95, 1964.

KOHN, B., & BRYDEN, M. P.: The effect of lysergic acid diethylamide on perception with stabilized images, Psychopharmacologia, **7**, 311–20, 1965.

KORNETSKY, C., HUMPHRIES, O., & EVARTS, E. V.: Comparison of psychological effects of certain centrally acting drugs in man, Arch. Neurol. & Psychiat., **77**, 318–24, 1957.

KRUS, D. M., & WAPNER, S.: Effect of lysergic acid diethylamide (LSD-25) on perception of part–whole relationships, J. Psychol., **48**, 87–95, 1959.

KURAMOCHI, H., & TAKAHASHI, R.: Psychopathology of LSD intoxication. Arch. Gen. Psychiat., **11**, 151–61, 1964.

LABARRE, W.: The Peyote Cult. Hamden, Conn., Shoestring Press, 1964.

LEBOVITS, B. Z., VISOTSKY, H. M., & OSTFELD, A. M.: LSD and JB-318: a comparison of two hallucinogens. II: An exploratory study, Arch. Gen. Psychiat. **2**, 390–407, 1960.

LEVINE, A., ABRAMSON, H. A., KAUFMAN, M. R., & MARKHAM, S.: Lysergic acid diethylamide (LSD–25). XVI: The effect on intellectual functioning as measured by the Wechsler-Bellevue Intelligence Scale, J. Psychol., **40**, 385–95, 1955.

LIEBERT, R. S., WAPNER, S., & WERNER, H.: Studies in the effects of lysergic acid diethylamide (LSD-25). Visual perception of verticality in schizophrenic and normal adults, Arch. Neurol. & Psychiat., **77**, 193–201, 1957.

LIEBERT, R. S., WERNER, H., & WAPNER, S.: Studies in the effect of lysergic acid diethylamide (LSD-25). Self and object size perception in schizophrenics and normal adults, Arch. Neurol & Psychiat., **79**, 580–4, 1958.

LINDEMANN, E., & Von FELSINGER, J. M.: Drug effects and personality theory, Psychopharmacologia, **2**, 69–92, 1961.

LING, T. M., & BUCKMAN, J.: The use of lysergic acid in individual psychotherapy, Proc. Roy. Soc. Med., **53**, 927–9, 1960.

LINTON, H. B., & LANGS, R. J.: Empirical dimensions of LSD-25 reaction, Arch. Gen. Psychiat., **10**, 469–85, 1964.

——— Subjective reactions to lysergic acid diethylamide (LSD-25), Arch. Gen. Psychiat., **6**, 352–68, 1962.

McGLOTHLIN, W. H., & COHEN, S.: The use of hallucinogenic drugs among college students, Am. J. Psychiat., **122**, 572–4, 1965.

McGLOTHLIN, W. H., COHEN, S., & McGLOTHLIN, M.S.: Short-term effects of LSD on anxiety, attitudes, and performance. J. Nerv. & Ment. Dis., **139**, 266–73, 1964.

MACLEAN, J. R., MACDONALD, D. C., BYRNE, U. P., and HUBBARD, A. M.: The use of LSD-25 in the treatment of alcoholism and other psychiatric problems, Quart. J. Stud. Alcohol, **22**, 34–5, 1961.

MACLEOD, M. Was dazed stranger the LSD suspect? New York Post, p. 6. April 14, 1966.

MALIS, J. L., BRODIE, D. A., & MORENO, O. M.: Drug effects on the behavior of self-stimulation monkeys. Fed. Proc. 19, 23, 1960.

MARTIN, A. J.: LSD (lysergic acid diethylamide) treatment of chronic psychoneurotic patients under day-hospital conditions, Intern. J. Soc. Psychiat., **3**, 188–95, 1957.

MEEHL, P.: Psychotherapy, Ann. Rev. Psychol., **6**, 357–78, 1955.

MEEHL, P. E.: Clinical versus Statistical Prediction. Minneapolis, University of Minnesota Press, 1954.

MONNIER, M.: Stimulants hallucinogènes, psychotoniques, et analeptiques du système nerveux central, XXIst Internat. Cong. Physiol. Sc., Buenos Aires, 149–58, 1959.

Nowlis, V., & Nowlis, H. H.: The description and analysis of mood. Ann. New York Acad. Sc., 64 (4), 343–55, 1956.

O'Reilly, P. O., & Funk, A.: LSD in chronic alcoholism. Canad. Psychiat. A. J., 258–61, 1964.

O'Reilly, P. O., & Reich, Genevieve: Lysergic acid and the alcoholic, Dis. Nerv. System, 23, 331–4, 1962.

Orsini, F., & Benda, P.: L'épreuve du dessin en miroir sous LSD-25, Ann. Med. Psychol., 118, 809–16, 1960.

Osmond, H., & Smythies, J.: Schizophrenia: A new approach, J. Ment. Sc., 98, 309–15, 1952.

Otis, L. S.: Dissociation and recovery of a response learned under the influences of chlorpromazine or saline, Science, 143, 1347–8, 1964.

Overton, D. A.: State-dependent or "dissociated" learning produced with phenobarbital, J. Comp. & Physiol. Psychol., 57, 3–12, 1964.

Purpura, D. P.: Electrophysiological analysis of psychotogenic drug action, A.M.A. Arch. Neurol. & Psychiat., 75, 122–31, 1956.

Ray, O. S., & Marrazzi, A. S.: Antagonism of behavioral effects of LSD by pre-treatment with chlorpromazine. Fed. Proc., 17, 24, 1960.

———— A quantifiable behavioral correlate of psychotogen and tranquilizer actions, Science, 133, 1705–6, 1961.

Resnick, O.: LSD-25 action in normal subjects treated with a monoamine oxidase inhibitor, Life Sc., 3, 1207–14, 1964.

———— Accentuation psychological effects of LSD-25 in normals with reserpine, Life Sc., 4, 1433–7, 1965.

Rinkel, M.: Experimentally induced psychoses in man, in Neuropharmacology, Transactions of the Second Conference, edited by H. A. Abramson. New York, Josiah Macy, Jr. Foundation, 1956.

———— The psychological aspects of the LSD psychosis, in Chemical Concepts of Psychosis, edited by M. Rinkel, and H. C. B. Denber. New York, McDowell Obelensky, 1958.

Rinkel, M., DeShon, H. J., Hyde, R. W., & Solomon, H. C.: Experimental schizophrenia-like symptoms, Am. J. Psychiat., 108, 572–8, 1952.

Robinson, J. T., Davies, L. S., Sack, E. L. N. S., & Morrissey, J. D.: A controlled trial of abreaction with lysergic acid diethylamide (LSD-25), Brit. J. Psychiat., 109, 46–53, 1963.

Rogers, C. R., & Dymond, Rosalind: Psychotherapy and personality change. Chicago, University of Chicago Press, 1954.

Rolo, A., Krinsky, L. W., Abramson, H. A., and Goldfarb, L.: Multitherapist interviews utilizing LSD, J. Psychol., 58, 237–9, 1964.

Sandison, R. A.: Psychological aspects of the LSD treatment of the neuroses, J. Ment. Sc. 100, 508–15, 1954.

Sandison, R. A., Spencer, A. M., & Whitelaw, J. D. A.: The therapeutic value of lysergic acid diethylamide in mental illness, J. Ment. Sc., 100, 491–507, 1954.

Sandison, R. A., & Whitelaw, J. D. A.: Further studies in the therapeutic value of lysergic acid diethylamide in mental illness, J. Ment. Sc., 103, 332–43, 1957.

Savage, C.: LSD transcendence and the new beginning, J. Nerv. & Ment. Dis., 135, 425–39, 1962.

Savage, C., Fadiman, J., Mogar, R., & Allen, Mary: Process and outcome variables in psychedelic (LSD) therapy. Unpublished MS, 1965.

Savage, C., & Stolaroff, M. J.: Clarifying the confusion regarding LSD-25, J. Nerv. & Ment. Dis., 140, 218–21, 1965.

Schachter, S.: The interaction of cognitive and physiological determinants of emotional state, in Psychobiological Approaches to Social Behavior, edited by P. H. Leiderman and D. Shapiro, Stanford University Press, 1965.

SCHAFER, R.: Psychoanalytic interpretation in Rorschach Testing. New York, Grune and Stratton, 1954.

SHEATZ, G. C., & BOGDANSKI, D. F.: Differential effect of LSD upon habituating and extinguishing evoked responses, J. Neuropsychiat. 5, 585–92, 1964.

SHERWOOD, J. N., STOLAROFF, M. J., & HARMAN, W. W.: The psychedelic experience—a new concept in psychotherapy, J. Neuropsychiat., 4, 69–80, 1962.

SILVERSTEIN, A. B., & KLEE, G. D.: The effect of lysergic acid diethylamide on digit span, J. Clin. & Exper. Psychopathol., 21, 11–14, 1960.

—— Effect of lysergic acid diethylamide (LSD-25) on intellectual functions, Arch. Neurol. & Psychiat., 80, 477–80, 1958.

—— The effect of lysergic acid diethylamide on dual pursuit performance, J. Clin. & Exper. Psychopathol., 21, 300–3, 1960.

SLATER, P. E., MORIMOTO, K., and HYDE, R. W.: The effect of group administration upon symptom formation under LSD, J. Nerv. & Ment. Dis., 125, 312–15, 1957.

SLOTKIN, J. A.: The Peyote Religion: A study in Indian–White Relations. Glencoe, The Free Press, 1956.

SMART, R. G., & STORM, T.: The efficacy of LSD in the treatment of alcoholism, Quart. J. Stud. Alcohol, 25, 333–8, 1964.

SMITH, C. M.: A new adjunct to the treatment of alcoholism: The hallucinogenic drugs, Quart. J. Stud. Alcohol, 19, 406–17, 1958.

—— Some reflections on the possible therapeutic effects of the hallucinogens, Quart. J. Stud. Alcohol, 20, 292–301, 1959.

—— Exploratory and controlled studies of lysergide in the treatment of alcoholism, Quart. J. Stud. Alcohol 25, 742–7, 1964.

SPENCER, A. M.: Permissive group therapy with LSD, Brit. J. Psychiat., 109, 37–45, 1963.

STAUDT, V., & ZUBIN, J.: A biometric evaluation of the somatotherapies in schizophrenia, Psychol. Bull. 54, 171–96, 1957.

STEIN, L.: Self selected brain stimulation reward threshold modified by drugs, Fed. Proc., 19, 264, 1960.

STOLL, W. A.: Lysergsäure diathylamid, ein Phantastikum aus der Mutterkorngruppe, Schweiz. Arch. Neurol. u. Psychiat., 60, 279–323, 1947.

—— Rorschach-Versuche unter Lysergsäure-Diathylamid-Wirkung, Rorschachiana, 1, 249–70, 1952.

STORM, T., & SMART, R. G.: Dissociation: A possible explanation of some features of alcoholism and implications for its treatment. Quart. J. Stud. Alcohol, 26, 111–15, 1965.

Subcommittee on Narcotics Addiction: The dangerous drug problem. New York Med., 22, 3–8, 1966.

TAESCHLER, M., WEIDMAN, H., & CERLETTI, A.: Die Wirkung von LSD auf die Reaktionszeiten bei einer bedingten Fluchtreaktion und im Analgesietest, Helvet. physiol. et pharmacol. acta, 18, 43–9, 1960.

TENENBAUM, B.: Group therapy with LSD-25, Dis. Nerv. System, 22, 459–62, 1961.

UNGER, S. M.: LSD and psychotherapy: A bibliography of the English-language literature, Psychedelic Rev., 1, 442–9, 1964.

—— Mescaline, LSD psilocybin, and personality change, Psychiatry, 26, 111–25, 1963.

VAN DUSEN, W., WILSON, W., MINERS, W., & HOOK, H.: Treatment of alcoholism with lysergide, prepublication abstract, Quart. J. Stud. Alcohol, 27, 534, 1966.

VANGGAARD, T.: Indications and counter-indications for LSD treatment. Acta psychiat. scandinav., **40**, 427–37, 1965.

WALLERSTEIN, R. S.: Hospital Treatment of Alcoholism: A Comparative, Experimental Study. New York, Basic Books, 1957.

WAPNER, S., & KRUS, D. M.: Effects of lysergic acid diethylamide, and differences between normals and schizophrenics on the Stroop Color Word Test, J. Neuropsychiat., **2**, 76–81, 1960.

WECKOWICZ, T. E.: The effect of lysergic acid diethylamide (LSD) on size constancy, Canad. Psychiat. A. J., **4**, 255–9, 1959.

WEINTRAUB, W., SILVERSTEIN, A. B., & KLEE, G. D.: The effect of LSD on the associative processes, J. Nerv. & Ment. Dis., **128**, 409–14, 1959.

WHITAKER, L. H.: Lysergic acid diethylamide in psychotherapy. Part I: Clinical aspects, M. J. Australia, **1**, 5–8, 1964a.

——— Lysergic acid diethylamide in psychotherapy. Part II. Results M. J. Australia, **1**, 36–41, 1964b.

WIKLER, A., ROSENBERG, D. E., HAWTHORNE, D. J., & CASSIDY, T. M.: Age and effect of LSD-25 on pupil size and kneejerk threshold, Psychopharmacologia, **7**, 44–56, 1965.

Appendix A

FOLLOW-UP QUESTIONNAIRE–DRINKING HISTORY

NAME: ....

AGE: ....

NUMBER OF YEARS OF SCHOOL: ....

PRESENT OCCUPATION: ....

DATE OF INTERVIEW: ....

I. TREATMENT HISTORY

  1. What contact have you had with clinic before? ....
     (obtain dates or period, nature of contact)

  2. Have you had any contact with other treatment facilities because of, or about your drinking?
     Private physician or psychiatrist? ....
     Clinic other than Brookside? ....
     A.A.? ....

  3. In the past year, for how much of the time have you been keeping up a relationship with some agency or other that deals with alcoholics? (Let patient volunteer, then ask to check closest.)

Not at all	Six months ....
Less than a month	Seven months ....
One month	Eight months ....
Two months	Nine months ....
Four months	Ten months ....
Five months	All year ....

II. DRINKING HISTORY

  1. Would you go through your drinking experiences in the past year, from a year ago to-day till the present time? Give as much detail about dates, time, circumstances, and so on as you possibly can.

  2. How often during the last year did you have one or more drinks?

.... not at all	.... three times a week
.... one to twelve times during the year	.... four times a week
.... once a week	.... five times a week
.... twice a week	.... daily

  3. During the past year, did you have as many as 3 or 4 drinks or any on any one occasion? ....

4. How often during the last year did you get drunk ....
drink enough so your speech and general behavior was definitely affected?

.... not at all   .... three times a week
.... one to twelve times during the year   .... four times a week
.... two or three times a month   .... five times a week
.... once a week   .... daily
.... twice a week

5. How often in the past year have you done any of the following:

	FRE-QUENTLY	SOME-TIMES	NEVER
(a) Neglected your meals while drinking	....	....	....
(b) Drunk just for the effect of the alcohol	....	....	....
(c) Taken a drink first thing in the morning	....	....	....
(d) Got drunk on a work day	....	....	
(e) Not been able to remember some of the things that happened while you were drinking	....	....	....
(f) Stayed drunk for several days in a row	....	....	....

6. What was your usual drink in the past year? ....
What else did you drink? ....

7. Where did you do most of your drinking the past year? ....
.... Any place else? ....

8. Whom did you do most of your drinking with? ....

9. What usually brought about these periods of drinking? ....

10. How much, in the past year, when you were not drinking, did you think about drinking and wish you had a drink? Just on the average.

.... all the time
.... every day, off and on
.... several times a week
.... once a week
.... two or three times a month
.... one–twelve times a year
.... not at all

III. ABSTINENCE

1. Have you had any periods of complete abstinence in the past year? ....

2. What was the longest period? (Get approximate dates, estimate of duration.) ....

3. What made you stay away from drinking in that period? Anything else? ....

4. Why did you begin drinking again? Any other reasons? ....

5. What other periods of abstinence did you have? (Get approximate dates and duration; ask about factors which brought about each period and reasons for terminating it.) ....
....

IV. DRUGS

1. Have you used any drugs in the past year? *If yes*, what did you use? ....
....
Why did you use these drugs? ....

2. Have you used any tranquilizers, or phenobarbital or sleeping pills, or any medicines of that sort? What? ....
Why? .... When? ....

V. PHYSICAL AND EMOTIONAL SYMPTOMS

1. Have you seen a doctor for any reason in the past year? ....
When? ....
For what reason? ....
For how long? ....

2. Have you taken medication of any kind in the past year? ....
What? ....
For what reason? ....
For how long? ....

3. Have you in the past year suffered from any of these conditions?

	FRE-QUENTLY	SOME-TIMES	NEVER
(a) dizzy spells	....	....	....
(b) palpitations or thumping in your heart	....	....	....
(c) rashes or other skin disorders	....	....	....
(d) cough (without a cold)	....	....	....
(e) shaking or trembling	....	....	....
(f) irritability	....	....	....
(g) inability to sleep	....	....	....
(h) anxiety for no apparent reason	....	....	....
(i) depression	....	....	....
(j) excessive sweating	....	....	....
(k) inability to concentrate	....	....	....
(l) severe headache	....	....	....
(m) diarrhea	....	....	
(n) nervousness in places like an elevator or tunnels	....	....	....
(o) stomach or intestinal pains	....	....	....
(p) great restlessness	....	....	....
(q) feelings of hopelessness	....	....	....
(r) indigestion or heartburn	....	....	....
(s) losing your temper	....	....	....
(t) asthma attacks	....	....	....
(u) constipation	....	....	....
(v) nausea	....	....	....
(w) great fatigue, for no apparent reason	....	....	....
(x) loss of appetite	....	....	....

4. Can you tell me your approximate weight at the present time? ....

VI. RESIDENTIAL MOBILITY

1. Where do you live now? ....
2. How many times have you moved in the past year? ....

103

3. Would you please tell me about each place you lived? When you lived there, address, whom you lived with, and your reason for moving?

ADDRESS	DATE	TYPE OF DWELLING	ALONE IF NOT, WITH WHOM?	REASON FOR MOVING

VII. OCCUPATIONAL HISTORY

1. Are you employed now? *If yes*, where do you work? ....
   What kind of work do you do? ....

2. How long have you been in this job? ....

3. What other jobs have you had in the past year? ....

DATE	TYPE OF JOB	WAGES OR SALARY	REASON FOR LEAVING

4. Have you been unemployed at any time in the past year? ....
   When? .... For how long? ....

5. Have you received any financial or other assistance from friends, relatives, or social agencies in the past year? .... *If yes*, what agency? ....
   ....
   About how much assistance? ....

6. How do you feel about the job you have now? ....
   ....

7. Would you say you are
   5. Very well satisfied ....
   4. Fairly satisfied ....
   3. Neutral ....
   2. Rather dissatisfied ....
   1. Very dissatisfied ....
   with your job.

8. What effect has drinking had on your job? ....
   ....

VIII. RELATIONSHIP WITH FELLOW-WORKERS AND EMPLOYERS

1. Are there any people directly under your supervision? ....
   If yes, how many? ....
2. How do you get along with them? ....
3. How do you feel about your boss? ....
4. Do you think you will stay in this job? ....
   5. Why? ....

IX. MARRIAGE AND FAMILY

1. Are you married now? ....

104

1(a) *If yes,* are you living with your wife at the present time? ....
Before coming into the clinic? ....

1(b) *If no to 1a,* have you lived together at any time in the past year? ....
If no to 1b, go to question 2.
If yes to 1a, how would you say you and your wife got along together
in the past year? ....

2. How would you describe your relations with your wife in the past year?
Excellent ....
Generally satisfactory ....
Indifferent ....
Generally unsatisfactory ....
Very satisfactory ....

3. Do you fight much? ....
What about? ....

4. About how often?
Never ....
Once in a while, say once a month ....
Once in a while, say once a week ....
Every day ....

5. Who handles the money?
I do, exclusively ....
I do, but I consult with her ....
She does, but we talk it over ....
She does, exclusively ....

6. Did you ever in the past year:

	FRE-QUENTLY	SOME-TIMES	NEVER
Wash dishes	....	....	....
Help with the shopping	....	....	....
Work on the house	....	....	....
Do the cleaning	....	....	....
Visit friends together	....	....	....
Go to a movie together	....	....	....
Have dinner out together	....	....	....
Go to clubs together	....	....	....

6(a) Is there anything else you do together? ....
What? ....

X. FRIENDS AND NEIGHBORS

1. How much of your time did you spend at home (in your room, etc.) in
the past year? ....
Almost never go out in the evening ....
Go out maybe one evening a month ....
Go out maybe two or three times a month ....
Go out maybe three or four evenings a week ....
Go out almost every evening ....

2. What do you do when you go out? ....

3. What do you do when you stay in? ....

4. About how many regular companions do you have (people that you see almost every week to go out, or meet some place, visit, or who visit you) in the past year?

No one ....   Four or five ....

One ....   Five to ten ....

Two or three ....   More than ten ....

4(a) How do you know them?

Old acquaintances ....   Neighbors ....

Drinking companions ....   Workmates ....

Belong to same clubs ....

5. How many people are there that you kept touch with regularly in the past year—who always knew roughly how you were, and whom you knew about?

No one ....   Four or five ....

One ....   Five to ten ....

Two or three ....   More than ten ....

6. Who would you say were your closest friends? ....

7. How long has it been since you saw each other? ....

8. Do you ever see your neighbors socially? ....
How often?

Never ....   Once per week ....

One to twelve times per year ....   Two to six times per week ....

Two to three times per month ....   Daily ....

Where? ....

8(a) How do you get along with your neighbors generally? ....
....

9. Do you ever see anybody from work off the job? ....
How often?

Never ....   Once per week ....

One to twelve times per year ....   Two to six times per week ....

Two to three times per month ....   Daily ....

Where? ....

10. Did you see any of your relatives in the past year?

Never ....   Once per week ....

One to twelve times per year ....   Two to six times per week ....

Two to three times per month ....   Daily ....

Where? ....

When? ....

11. Did you write to any friends, relatives, etc., in the past year? ....
How often?

Never ....   Once per week ....

One to twelve times per year ....   Two to six times per week ....

Two to three times per month ....   Daily ....

To whom? ....

XI. RELATIVES

    1. Are either of your parents living? ....

    2. *If yes,* how often did you see them in the past year? ....

    3. How did you get along with them in the past year? ....

    4. Any sisters or brothers? ....

    5. *If yes,* did you see them in the past year (how often)? ....

    6. How did you get along with them in the past year? ....

    7. *If married,* did you see any of your in-laws in the past year? ....
       How often? ....

    8. How did you get along with them in the past year? ....

XII. ACTIVITIES (FORMAL)

    1. Do you belong to any clubs or organizations? ....
       (a) Which ones? ....
       (b) How long have you been a member? ....
       (c) Did you hold any office? ....
       (d) How often have you attended in the past year? ....

XIII. INCARCERATIONS

    1. Have you been in jail at all in the past year? ....
       (a) How many times? ....
       (b) How long each time? ....
       (c) When was this? ....
       (d) Reason? ....

    2. Have you been fined at all in the past year? ....
       (a) For what reason? ....

Following is a list of statements a person might make about himself. Indicate for each statement whether *you* would make that statement about *yourself.*

I WOULD SAY THAT	YES	NO
1. I am generally dissatisfied with the kind of person I am.	....	....
2. My friends and family think I am quite intelligent, but I'm really not.	....	....
3. I am not the kind of person I would like my family and friends to think I am.	....	....
4. My friends and family think I work hard but I really don't.	....	....
5. I am usually not satisfied with the impression that I make on others.	....	....
6. Friends and family think I am ambitious, but I'm really not.	....	....
7. I am not the kind of person that I would really like to be.	....	....

8. Friends and family think I am a very honest person, but I'm not as honest as they think. ....

9. I sometimes feel that the best solution for my problems would be to be dead. ....

10. Friends and family think I am a very kind person, but I don't think so. ....

11. I am not satisfied with my ability to get along with other people. ....

12. I am not living up to the expectations of my family and friends. ....

13. Family and friends think I am very generous, but I don't think so. ....

14. I am not the kind of person I think family and friends expect me to be. ....

15. I usually do not agree with what I think other people think of me. ....

Now here are a few statements that a person's family and friends might make about him. Which of these do you think *your* family and friends would make about *you*?

I THINK THEY WOULD SAY THAT   YES   NO

1. They are usually displeased with what I do and the way I do it. ....

2. My performance is usually below what they think it should be. ....

3. I don't try hard enough to do a good job. ....

4. I am not the kind of person they would like me to be. ....

5. I am not living up to their standards. ....

6. I could do better in most things than I actually do. ....

Can you give me the names of five people who are likely to know, during the next year, how you are getting along?

NAME	ADDRESS
....	....
....	....
....	....
....	....
....	....

Do you have any objection to our getting in touch with them later on to see how you are doing? ....

Appendix B

TABLE I

CHANGES IN DRINKING BEHAVIOR: THE ANALYSIS OF VARIANCE FOR THE DIFFERENCES
BETWEEN THE THREE TREATMENT GROUPS IN THE PRE- AND POST-TREATMENT PERIODS
FOR NUMBER OF DRINKING OCCASIONS

Source	Degrees of freedom	Mean square	F	P
Periods	1	1760.4	18.6	<0.001
Groups	2	296.6	3.14	>0.05
Periods $\times$ groups	2	18.8	0.20	>0.05
Error	54	94.4		
TOTAL	59			

TABLE II

CHANGES IN DRUNKENNESS OCCURRENCES: THE ANALYSIS OF VARIANCE FOR THE DIF-
FERENCES BETWEEN THE THREE TREATMENT GROUPS IN THE PRE- AND POST-TREAT-
MENT PERIODS FOR NUMBER OF DRUNKENNESS OCCASIONS

Source	Degrees of freedom	Mean square	F	P
Periods	1	238.1	5.30	<0.05
Groups	2	117.9	2.63	>0.05
Periods $\times$ groups	2	46.5	1.0	>0.05
Error	54	44.9		
TOTAL	59			

TABLE III

CONVICTIONS FOR DRUNKENNESS IN THE PRE- AND
FIRST POST-TREATMENT PERIODS

Group	Pre-treatment	First-post-treatment
Control	2	1
LSD	8	4
Ephedrine	4	6

TABLE IV

PSYCHOLOGICAL CHANGES: MEANS FOR THE THREE TREATMENT
GROUPS IN NEUROTICISM (N) AND EXTROVERSION (E)

	Score	Pre-treatment	Post-treatment
Control	N	33.2	28.8
	E	20.9	23.1
LSD	N	38.6	30.8
	E	20.1	20.1
Ephedrine	N	28.9	26.7
	E	28.0	26.0

TABLE V

MEAN RORSCHACH SCORES FOR (R), (M), (C), AND
(K) FOR THE THREE TREATMENT GROUPS

Control	Pre-treatment	Post-treatment
R	15.7	22.3
M	1.6	2.6
C	4.3	3.1
K	9.0	4.0
LSD		
R	20.0	21.4
M	1.4	2.1
C	3.4	4.0
K	6.0	4.0
Ephedrine		
R	20.9	21.4
M	2.0	2.1
C	4.8	3.8
K	12.0	4.0

TABLE VI

CLINICAL JUDGMENTS OF RORSCHACH CHANGES FROM THE PRE-
TREATMENT TO THE POST-TREATMENT PERIOD

	Same	More	Less	Uncertain
		Range of emotions		
Control	6	2	3	
Ephedrine	6	1	2	
LSD	6	3	1	
		Indications of anxiety		
Control	5	0	5	
Ephedrine	4	0	5	
LSD	3	2	5	
		Amount of internal conflict		
Control	5	0	5	
Ephedrine	6	0	3	
LSD	4	2	4	
		Amount of repression		
Control	5	1	4	
Ephedrine	3	4	2	
LSD	3	2	5	
		Degree of self-acceptance		
Control	7	3	0	
Ephedrine	7	1	1	
LSD	7	3	0	
		Indication of guilt feelings		
Control	4	0	5	1
Ephedrine	3	0	2	4
LSD	2	0	3	5

TABLE VII

Q-SORT MOVEMENT INDEX MEANS

Group	Index	1 G-D	2 F-B	3 H-A	4 J-I	5 E-B	6 F-C	7 C-B	8 F-E
No drug control	M_D	0.030	0.162	0.103	0.274	0.070	0.149	0.013	0.092
	SE_{MD}	0.145	0.146	0.108	0.097	0.093	0.124	0.077	0.096
	P	N.S.	N.S.	N.S.	<0.03	N.S.	N.S.	N.S.	N.S.
A	N	10	10	10	10	10	10	10	10
L.S.D.	M_D	0.134	0.047	0.092	0.204	0.071	0.097	0.144	0.024
	SE_{MD}	0.088	0.102	0.101	0.124	0.074	0.074	0.082	0.065
	P	N.S.	N.S.	N.S.	N.S.	N.S.	N.S.	N.S.	N.S.
B	N	9	9	9	9	9	9	9	9
Ephedrine control	M_D	0.202	0.273	0.231	0.076	0.182	0.179	0.056	0.091
	SE_{MD}	0.169	0.163	0.147	0.128	0.159	0.131	0.067	0.090
	P	N.S.	N.S.	N.S.	N.S.	N.S.	N.S.	N.S.	N.S.
C	N	8	8	8	8	8	8	8	8

TABLE VIII

DIFFERENCES BETWEEN GROUPS ($M_{DA} - M_{DB}$, ETC.) ON MOVEMENT INDICES

Group	Index	1 G-D	2 F-B	3 H-A	4 J-I	5 E-B	6 F-C	7 C-B	8 F-E
A–B	M_A–M_B	0.164	0.209	0.011	0.070	0.141	0.052	0.157	0.068
	SE_{MD}	0.175	0.182	0.149	0.155	0.120	0.148	0.134	0.118
	P	N.S.	N.S.	N.S.	N.S.	N.S.	N.S.	N.S.	N.S.
B–C	M_B–M_C	0.336	0.226	0.139	0.128	0.111	0.276	0.088	0.115
	SE_{MD}	0.185	0.188	0.175	0.179	0.169	0.145	0.106	0.109
	P	<0.10	N.S.	N.S.	N.S.	N.S.	<0.10	N.S.	N.S.
A–C	M_A–M_C	0.172	0.435	0.128	0.198	0.252	0.328	0.069	0.183
	SE_{MD}	0.222	0.219	0.178	0.160	0.176	0.181	0.103	0.134
	P	N.S.	<0.10	N.S.	N.S.	N.S.	<0.10	N.S.	N.S.

TABLE IX

NUMBER OF MARRIED PATIENTS LIVING WITH WIVES

	Pre-treatment	Post-treatment
LSD	2	1
Ephedrine	6	5
Control	3	4

TABLE X

NUMBER OF PATIENTS WHO CHANGED RESIDENCE

	Pre-treatment	Post-treatment
LSD	8	6
Ephedrine	3	4
Control	3	2

Index

ABRAMSON, H. A.: on the Jungians and the Freudians and the psychological use of LSD, 16; and LSD in psychoanalysis, 55; and LSD in psychotherapy, 14; and LSD treatment of alcoholism, 44; on patient–therapist interaction, 16; on suicide and the LSD user, 9. See also Jarvik, M. E.; Levine, A.; Rolo, A.

Abramson, H. A. et al.: on character of LSD experience, 23; and LSD and spatial-relations tests, results, 19

Abramson, H. A., M. E. Jarvik, and M. W. Hirsch, on verbal reaction time, effect of LSD, 19

Abramson, H., M. Jarvick, M. Kaufman, C. Kornetsky, A. Levine, and M. Wagner, on LSD treatment and placebo reaction, 48

Abramson, H., M. Jarvik, A. Levine, M. R. Kaufman, and M. Hirsch, on LSD treatment and placebo reactors, 48

Addiction, possibility with LSD, 11

Addiction Research Foundation, investigation on LSD and alcoholism

drinking behavior: and family, employment, and social stability, 81, 88; psychological changes from 76–80, 86–8

follow-up questionnaire, App. A

methods: administration of LSD and ephedrine, 63–5; the alcoholic patients and their assignment to treatment groups, 60–2; controls and double-blind procedures, effectiveness, 68–9; empirical and methodological bases for, 50–60; evaluation procedures before drug administration, 63; post-treatment evaluation and follow-up, 65–6; psychological test administration, 66–8; treatment setting, 62

results, 70–81, App. B

shortcomings of study, 85

Alcoholics Anonymous, 45

Alcoholism: therapy as effective without LSD, 85–5; and use of LSD in Saskatchewan, 53–4, 55. See also Addiction Research Foundation investigation

Allen, Mary, See Savage, C.

Alpert, Richard, on indiscriminate use of hallucinogens, 13

Arendsen-Hein, G. W., LSD treatment of criminal psychopaths, 33

Armstrong, J. J. See Ball, J. R.; Gibbons, R. J.

Aronson, H. and G. D. Klee, LSD and maze test, 19

Aronson, H., A. B. Silverstein, and G. W. Klee, on time judgment, effect of LSD, 20

BACH, S. A. See Baldwin, M.

Bacon, S. D., improvement rates, under all existing therapies, 3

Baker, E. F. W. on anxiety effect of LSD, 31; on non-psychotic patients treated with LSD, 29

Baldwin, M., S. A. Lewis, and S. A. Bach, on effects of LSD after cerebral ablation, 18

Ball, J. R. and J. J. Armstrong, on LSD treatment of patients with sexual perversions, 32–3

Benda, P. See Orsini, F.

Benda, P. and F. Orsini, on time judgment, effects of LSD, 20

Bender, L., G. Faretra, and R. L. Cobrini, on the use of LSD with psychotic children, 28–9

Benedetti, G., LSD treatment with alcoholics, 44n

Bennett, Richard, 65n

Bercel, N. A. et al., on LSD as psychotomimetic drug, 6, 7

Blewett, D. B. See Chwelos, N.

Blough, D. S., on response rates for

115

positive reinforcers and LSD (animal studies), 20
Boardman, W. K., S. Goldstone, and W. T. Lhamon, on time judgment, effects of LSD, 20
Boeri, G. *See* Giberti, F.
Bogdanski, D. F. *See* Sheatz, G. C.
Brehm, J. W. and A. R. Cohen, on behavioral commitment, effect on attitudes, 36
Brodie, D. A. *See* Malis, J. L.
Bryden, M. P. *See* Kohn, B.
Buckman, J. *See* Ling, T. M.
Bunnell, S. on biochemical effects of LSD, 17; on the lethal dose of LSD, 8; on tolerance to LSD, 11
Busch, A. K. and W. C. Johnson; first report of the use of LSD in psychotherapy, 14
Butterworth, A. T., on LSD treatment of patients, 32
Byrne, U. P. *See* MacLean, J. R.

CARLSON, V. R., on visual perception, effects of LSD, 19
Cassidy, T. M. *See* Wikler, A.
Cerletti, A. *See* Taeschler, M.
Chandler, A. and Hartman: on LSD and the follow-up period, 9; and LSD as part of a psychoanalytically oriented program, result, 30–1; and LSD studies with alcoholics, 43, 50, 56, 90–1
Chwelos, N. *et al.*: on importance of stimuli in LSD experiments, 92; and LSD, amount used, 91; and LSD and self-acceptance, 87; and LSD studies with alcoholics, 43, 48, 50, 51, 56, 82, 84; and refinements of LSD methodology, 84; and social–psychological factors and LSD, 26
Cobrini, R. L. *See* Bender, L.
Cohen, A. R. *See* Brehm, J. W.
Cohen, S.: on alcoholics, and the use of peyote, 4; on LSD and therapist involvement, 13; on non-medical use of LSD, 10; on psychoses, complications from non-medical use of LSD, 12; on suicide and use of LSD, 9. *See also* Eisner, B. G.; McGlothlin, W. H.
Cohen, S. and K. S. Ditman, on black-market sale of hallucinogenic drugs, 10; on dangers of LSD, 8;

and long LSD series, 11; on psychotic complications, from non-medical use of LSD, 12; on psychological dependence on LSD, 11; on rate of psychoses in LSD therapy, 12
Cohen, S., L. Fichman, and B. G. Eisner, on LSD and intelligence test results, 19

DAVIDSON, H. H. *See* Klopfer, B.
Davies, L. S. *See* Robinson, J. T.
Deshon, H. J. *See* Rinker, M.
Ditman, K. on psychotic complications, from non-medical use of LSD, 12
Ditman, K. *See* Cohen S.
Ditman, K., M. Hayman, and J. Whittlesey: on LSD effects in non-treatment setting, 35–6; and LSD experience and mystics, 36; and LSD in non-treatment setting with alcoholics, results, 43; and LSD treatment, outcome, 41
Ditman, K. and J. R. B. Whittlesey, on character of the LSD experience, 22
Dreikurs, E. *See* Bercel, N. A.
Dymond, Rosalind. *See* Rogers, C. R.

EISNER, B. G. *See* Cohen, S.
Eisner, B. G. and S. Cohen: on LSD and alcoholism, and selection of doses, 90–1; and LSD, therapist's personal experience with, 36; and LSD treatment of alcoholics, 43, 50, 51, 56; and LSD treatment of neurotic patients, 32
Ends, E. J. and C. W. Page: Haigh–Butler Q Sort, before and after therapy, 68; self and ideal changes in psychotherapy, 78, 79
Evarts, E. V. *See* Kornetsky, C.
Ewald, A. T. *See* Abramson, H. A.; Jarvik, M. E.
Eysenck, H. J.: criticism of research on treatment methods, 43; neuroticism, extroversion, and character disorders, 49; review of studies of improvement in neurotics, 41

FADIMAN, J. *See* Savage, C.
Faretra, G. *See* Bender, L.
Festinger, L., on behavioral commitment, effect on attitudes, 36
Fichman, L. *See* Cohen, S.

Fink, H. *See* Haas, M.
Fontana, A. E., on LSD treatment of psychoneurotics, 33
Foulds, G.: on lack of controls in studies of new treatments, 48; on low scientific standards in clinical trials of new drugs, 43
Freedman, D. X., on biochemical effects of LSD, 17
Funk, A. *See* O'Reilly, P. O.

GIBBINS, R. J. AND J. D. ARMSTRONG: on average gains of abstinence without LSD, 85; and treatment for alcoholism, 62
Giberti, F., L. Gregoretti, and G. Boeri, on LSD treatment of neurotics, 33
Glick, B. and R. Margolis: on double-blind controlled and non-blind uncontrolled studies, 83; and improvement rates, double-blind controlled and non-blind uncontrolled studies, 48; on low scientific standards in the clinical trials of new drugs, 43
Goldfarb, L. *See* Rolo, A.
Goldstone, S. *See* Boardman, W. K.
Gregoretti, L. *See* Giberti, F.
Griener, T., on single-blind and double-blind drug trials, 83

HAIGH–BUTLER Q SORT, 68, 78–80
Haas, M., H. Fink, and G. Hartfelder, on double-blind trials, criticism of, 49
Harman, W. W. *See* Sherwood, J. W.
Hartfelder, G. *See* Haas, M.
Hartman, A. M., on the Jungians and Freudians and the psychological use of LSD, 16
Hartman, A. M. *See* also Chandler, A.
Hartman, A. M. and L. E. Hollister, on color perception, effects of LSD, 19–20
Hawthorne, D. J. *See* Wikler, A.
Hayman, M. *See* Ditman, K.
Heiss-Sandler figure test, and LSD, 19
Hirsch, M. W. *See* Abramson, H. A.; Jarvik, M. E.
Hoffer, A.: on biochemical effects of LSD, 17; on hallucinogenic properties of adrenolutin and adrenochrome, 7; LSD treatment of alcoholics in Saskatchewan, 54; on suicide and the LSD user, 8
Hoffer, A. *See* also Chwelos, N.

Hofmann, A., hallucinogenic properties of LSD, discovery of, 6
Hollister, L. E. *See* Hartman A. M.
Honigfeld, G., on effect of LSD on speech, 19
Hook, H. *See* Van Dusen, W.
Hubbard, A. M. *See* MacLean, J. R.
Humphries, O. *See* Kornetsky, C.
Hyde, R. W. *See* Rinkel, M.; Slater, D. E.

INDIANS, NORTH AMERICAN, and the use of peyote, 4–5
International Federation for International Freedom, 13
Isbell, H., on character of LSD experience, 22

JACOBSEN, E., introduction of antabuse therapy, 3
Jarvik, M. E. *See* Abramson, H. A.
Jarvik, M. E., H. A. Abramson, and M. W. Hirsch, on LSD and memory test results, 19
Jarvik, M. E., *et al.*, on LSD and arithmetic test results, 19
Jensen, S. E., and R. Ramsay: LSD, amount used, 91; and LSD treatment of alcoholics, 44, 45–8, 50, 51, 56, 57; and large number in LSD study, 83
Johnson, G. H.: on LSD and alcoholics, results with four groups, 86; and LSD, therapeutic effectiveness of, 93
Johnson, W. C. *See* Busch, A. K.
Jones, Maxwell, on alcoholism and drug addiction clinics, 62
Joyce, C., on placebo reactors – neuroticism and extroversion, 49

KAUFMAN, M. R. *See* Abramson, H.; Levine, A.
Kelley, D. M. *See* Klopfer, B.
Key, B. J.: on effects of LSD on sensory transmissions, 17–18; and neurophysiological effects of LSD, 18
Killam, E. K. *See* Killam, K. F.
Killam, K. F. and E. K. Killam; on neurophysiological effects of LSD 18
Klee, G. D. *See* Aronson, H.; Weintraub, W.
Klee, G. W. *See* Aronson, H.; Silverstein, A. B.

Klopfer, B., D. M. Kelley, and H. H. Davidson, Rorschach scoring system, 67
Knowles, J. and C. Lucas: placebo reactors—neuroticism and extroversion, 49
Knudsen, K., on homicide following LSD, 10
Kohn, B. and M. P. Bryden, target stimulus, effects of LSD, result, 20
Kornetsky, C. See Abramson, H.
Kornetsky, C., O. Humphries, and E. V. Evarts, LSD and memory test results, 19
Krinsky, L. W. See Rolo, A.
Krus, D. M. See Wapner, S.
Krus, D. M., and S. Wapner: Heiss–Sandler figure test, effect of LSD, 19
Kuramochi, H. and R. Takahashi, LSD, obvious effects of, 90

LA BARRE, W., on LSD and therapist involvement, 13; and the Navajos' use of peyote, 5; on non-medical use of hallucinogenic drugs, 10; and peyote, use in Mexico, 4; peyote and alcohol, incompatibility of, 5; and pre-Columbian Mexico, use of peyote and mescal, 6
Langs, R. J. See Linton, H. B.
Leary, T., and indiscriminate use of hallucinogens, 13
Lebovits, B. Z., H. M. Vistotsky, and A. M. Ostfeld, on character of LSD experience, 22
Levine, A. See Abramson, H.
Levine, A., et al., on LSD and intelligence test results, 19
Levinson, Mrs. Toby, 67n
Lewis, S. A. See Baldwin, M.
Lhamon, W. T. See Boardman, W. K.
Liebert, R. S., S. Wapner, and H. Werner, visual perception, effects of LSD, 19
Liebert, R. S., H. Werner, and S. Wapner, visual perception, effects of LSD, 19
Lindemann, E. and J. M. Von Felsinger, on complexity of effects of any drug, 15
Ling, T. M. and J. Buckman, results of LSD-aided psychotherapy, 31-2
Linton, H. B. and R. J. Langs: lack of follow-up procedures, 9; on LSD

reaction vs. natural schizophrenic disorders, 7; on normal reaction to LSD, 7; and subjective effects of LSD, 20-1
Lucas, C. See Knowles, J.
LSD (lysergic acid diethylamide): and alcoholics, early reports of use, 3; and alteration in response patterns, 25-6; and biochemical theory of schizophrenia, early studies, 7; and dangers of, 8-13; direction of future research with, 90-3; discovery of, 6; early use of, 4-5; early psychiatric use of, 6-8; effects on family, employment, and social stability, 57-8; effects on personality in alcoholics, 55-7; effect on sensory transmission, 17-18; and fluency of response and reaction time, 19; and general sympathetic activation, 23-4; and intelligence test results, 18-19; low toxicity of, 8; and need for properly controlled experiments, 28, 30, 48-50; normal reaction to, 6-7; and objective test results, 18-19; and perceptual distortions, 24-5; and placebo effects, 48-9; "psychedelic," effect of, 7; and psychomotor task results, 19; as a psychotomimetic drug, 6; purposes of monograph, 3-4; social effects on alcoholics, 57-8; and suicide, 6, 8-10; therapist's experience with drug, 92; and visual perception, 19-20; weakness of research in. See also Alcoholic Research Foundation investigation

MACDONALD, D. C. See MacLean, J. R.
McGlothlin, M. S. See McGlothlin, W. H.
McGlothlin, W. H. and S. Cohen, on personality factors and the LSD experience, 26
McGlothlin, W. H., S. Cohen, and M. S. McGlothlin, LSD, positive attitude towards, and personality type, 36
MacLean, J. R. et al.: LSD, amount used, 91; and LSD, effect on personality of alcoholics, 56; and LSD and therapist participation, 92; and LSD treatment of alcoholics, pre- and post-treatment procedures, and results, 43, 44, 50-1, 57-8, 82, 90

natural schizophrenic disorders, 7; and normal reaction to LSD, 7

Robinson, J. T. *et al.*: LSD treatment outcome, 41; and patients randomly assigned to LSD or comparison group, 38–9

Rogers, C. R. and Rosalind Dymond, Haigh–Butler *Q* Sort, 68

Rolo, A. *et al.*, on the result of LSD treatment, 29–30

Rorschach test: administration of, 67–8; effect of LSD, 19; in evaluation of psychological changes, 76–8

Rosenberg, D. E. *See* Wikler, A.

SACK, E. L. N. S. *See* Robinson, J. T.

Saskatchewan Bureau on Alcoholism, on use of LSD on treatment of alcoholism, 53–4, 55

Sandison, R. A., on the abreactive qualities of LSD, 31

Sandison, R. A., A. M. Spencer, and J. D. A. Whitelaw, modification of therapeutic LSD procedure, 31

Sandison, R. A. and J. D. A. Whitelaw, results of LSD therapy, 31

Savage, C.: on LSD treatment with alcoholics, 44; and social stability, 58

Savage, C. *et al.*: on the importance of the total setting in psychological treatment, 15–16; on LSD, effects on values and behavior, 27; and LSD treatment, "psychedelic" orientation, 34–5, 36

Savage, C. and M. J. Stolaroff, on variations in therapy procedure, 27–8

Schachter, S.: on the importance of the total setting in psychological treatment, 15; on the physiological arousal produced by drugs, 23

Schafer, R., on human movement responses and personality, 67

Sheatz, G. C. and D. F. Bogdanski, LSD and Pavlovian conditioning of animals, 18

Sherwood, J. N., M. J. Stolaroff, and W. W. Harman, on LSD treatment, psychedelic orientation of, 33–4

Silverstein, A. B. *See* Aronson, H.; Weintraub, W.

Silverstein, A. B. and G. D. Klee: on LSD and intelligence tests, results, 19; and LSD and psychomotor tasks, results, 19

Slotkin, J. A.: on alcoholics, and the use of peyote, 4; and Navajos' use of peyote, 5; on non-addictive nature of peyote, 11; on peyote and alcohol, incompatibility of, 5

Slater, P. E., K. Morimoto, and R. W. Hyde, on importance of setting, 22

Smart, R. G. *See* Storm, T.

Smart, R. G. and T. Storm: on LSD therapy with alcoholics, length of follow-up periods, 9; on requirements for research into the efficacy of new treatment, 28

Smith, C. M.: on dangers of LSD, 8; and importance of stimuli in LSD experiments, 92; and LSD and alchoholism, results, 90; and LSD, doses used, 91; and LSD and therapist's participation, 92; and LSD treatment of alcoholics, 43, 48, 50, 51, 54, 56, 57, 82, 84; and LSD trials, defence of, 52; and no LSD experience before first study, 64; and psychopaths and psychotics least affected by LSD therapy, 92; and social–psychological factors and LSD, 26. *See also* Chwelos, N.

Smythies, J. *See* Hoffer A.; Osmond, H.

Solomon, H. C. *See* Rinkel, M.

Spencer, A. M., on use of LSD in group psychotherapy, 33. *See also* Sandison, R. A.

Stein, L., response rates for positive reinforcers and LSD (animal studies), 20

Stolaroff, M. J. *See* Savage C.; Sherwood, J. N.

Stoll, W. A.: on LSD treatment of mentally ill, 6; and Rorschach test, effect of LSD, 19

Storm, T. *See* Smart, R. G.

Storm, T. and R. G. Smart, on alcohol intoxication and memory loss, 25

Stroop color-word test and LSD, 19

Suicide, and LSD users, 6, 8–10

TAESCHLER, M., H. WEIDMAN, AND A. CERLETTI, on negative responses, and LSD, 20

Takahashi, R. *See* Kuramochi, H.

Tenenbaum, B., use of LSD in group psychotherapy, 33

Travis, L. E. *See* Bercel, N. A.

120

121